W9-AUD-701

Children's Communication Skills

Speech and language are fundamental to human development. Language is needed for both communication and thought, while education depends on the ability to understand and use language competently. Effective communication underpins social and emotional well-being.

Children's Communication Skills: From Birth to Five Years uses a clear format to set out the key stages of communication development in babies and young children. Its aim is to increase awareness in professionals working with children of what constitutes human communication and what communication skills to expect at any given stage. Illustrated throughout with real-life examples, this informative text addresses:

- normal development of verbal and non-verbal communication skills
- the importance of play in developing these skills
- developmental communication problems
- bilingualism, cognition and early literacy development
- working with parents of children with communication difficulties.

Features designed to make the book an easy source of reference include chapter summaries, age-specific skills tables, sections on warning signs that further help may be needed, and a glossary of key terms.

These practical guidelines on what to expect children to achieve and how to help them get there are based on a huge body of research in child language and communication development. *Children's Communication Skills: From Birth to Five Years* will be of great use to a wide range of professionals in training or working in health, education and social care: health visitors; general practitioners; community nurses; educational psychologists; early years educators; and speech and language therapists.

Belinda Buckley is a Paediatric Speech and Language Therapist.

Children's Communication Skills

From Birth to Five Years

Belinda Buckley

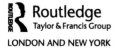

Routledge
Taylor & Francis Group

LONDON AND NEW YORK

First published 2003
by Routledge
11 New Fetter Lane, London EC4P 4EE

Simultaneously published in the USA and Canada
by Routledge
29 West 35th Street, New York, NY 10001

Transferred to Digital Printing 2004

Routledge is an imprint of the Taylor & Francis Group

© 2003 Belinda Buckley

Illustrations © 2003 Steve Rose

Typeset in Times by
Keystroke, Jacaranda Lodge, Wolverhampton

Printed in Great Britain by Biddles Ltd., King's Lynn, Norfolk

British Library Cataloguing in Publication Data
A catalogue record for this book is available from the British Library

Library of Congress Cataloging in Publication Data
Buckley, Belinda, 1965–
    Children's communication skills : from birth to five years / Belinda Buckley.
        p. cm.
    Includes bibliographical references (p.) and index.
    1. Interpersonal communication in children. 2. Nonverbal
    communication in children. I. Title.

    BF723.C57 .B78 2003
    401′.93—dc21   2002036931

ISBN 0–415–25993–2 (Hbk)
ISBN 0–415–25994–0 (Pbk)

For Rowan

Contents

Figures

Examples and case studies

Examples

Case studies

Tables

Key skills

Warning signs

Preface

The 'what' and 'how' of communication

The purpose of this book is to increase awareness in professionals working with babies and young children of what constitutes human communication and what communication skills to expect from birth to 5 years of age. Greater knowledge in these areas should lead to greater confidence among professionals in identifying those children having problems in developing their speech, language and communication. There is much evidence to support early intervention for babies and very young children with communication difficulties. Importantly, professionals need to know that they do not have to wait for a child to start talking before discussing their communication skills development with parents.

Essentially, all children are thought to have an innate predisposition to develop nonverbal and verbal communication skills. It is helpful to consider communication by asking the following two questions: what is it and how is it used? Answers to the first question include smiling, eye contact, gesture and language. Answers to the second question include expressing pleasure, signalling to other speakers that one has finished speaking, drawing another person's attention to an interesting toy and telling stories. The 'what' of communication emerges in all children but it is the socio-cultural and linguistic environment that plays a significant part in determining 'how' children use these skills. Cultures differ in this respect. There are differences between cultures regarding what is considered appropriate use of eye gaze between adults and children, regarding how smiling is used and which gestures are deemed appropriate. Within cultures, the context of the interaction determines how communication skills are used, as what is considered appropriate depends on the context. There are rules within cultures that determine what is and is not appropriate in terms of use of communication. Children learn these rules implicitly over the course of their development.

This book describes the 'what' of communication skills development in babies and children. Babbling, smiling, pointing, vocalizing, using words one at a time, combining words, understanding situations and understanding words are all communication skills and are universal. The rate of emergence of many of these skills occurs universally among children with normal communication skills development (Bates *et al.* in press). All babies babble around the same time, but the sounds they produce are influenced by the sounds of the language spoken around them. Smiling emerges universally around the same time in children, but children have to learn the cultural rules for using smiles in interaction with others. There has not been extensive research, however, into rates of emergence of the range of nonverbal and verbal communication skills cross-culturally and cross-linguistically.

This book also describes the 'how' of communication skills development, from a largely western, monolingual English-speaking perspective. Of course there are variations between western English-speaking children regarding how they use their communication skills – cultures and societies have never been static, and many western societies are becoming increasingly multicultural and multilingual. There is an intricate relationship between the 'what' and the 'how' of communication skills that necessitates a cautious approach towards applying information in this book to children for whom it is not culturally appropriate.

Analysing communication

Human communication involves a highly complex interplay of skills (such as language), mental processes (such as thinking about what somebody has said) and physical movements (such as hand gestures and facial expressions). For example, as you read the words on this page you might be aware of sounds in your environment such as cars passing by outside or of somebody sneezing. Although your ears might sense these sounds and transmit them to your brain, you are able to direct your attention to your reading, simultaneously filtering out environmental sounds (for a certain amount of time, anyway). The skills and processes central to reading (which at a minimum are control over one's focus of attention, and extracting meaning from written words) occur simultaneously.

It is helpful to analyse communication in terms of its component skills, processes and behaviours, in order to understand it better. When considering the development of communication skills in children, it is also helpful to draw links with related areas of development such as play and attention. Development of the various skills involved in communication occurs simultaneously in most children, relevant to their stage of development. For purposes of clarity, different aspects of communication (for example, understanding words, using words, using gestures) are discussed independently in Chapters 1 to 4. The format of these chapters is the same, and reflects the range of skills involved in communication and important related skills. However, every effort has been made to relate the various aspects of communication not only to each other, but also to related areas of development. It is important to keep in mind that the development of communication skills is inextricably linked to other areas of a child's development. Understanding a child's communication is one step towards understanding them as a whole child.

Use of examples

The book contains several examples of communication behaviours and child language. Most of these are from observations of a girl called Rowan during her early years. However, there are also examples from other children, some of whom are Rowan's friends.

Referring to significant adults

A book about the development of children's communication skills would be impossible to write without mention of the significant adults in children's lives. 'Significant adults' refers to parents and other main caregivers. Many children have more than one significant adult in their lives. The importance and value of each of these adults' contribution to any child's overall development, including that of their communication skills, is not in question. There is no direct or indirect intention in this book to express value for one gender over another, or to suggest that one relationship that a child has with one parent, or main caregiver, is more important, or valuable, than another. For purposes of readability and when discussing specific examples of communication between an adult and a child, the terms, 'mother', 'father', 'parent' and 'caregiver' have variously been used. More reference is made to interaction between mothers (i.e. rather than fathers and other caregivers) and babies in Chapter 1, as this covers the early weeks and months in a baby's life, which is usually spent in close contact with their mother.

Referring to children

Except in specific examples of communication involving boys, I have used 'she' when referring to children in this book. This is for purposes of clarity and consistency.

Tables outlining communication skills usually achieved by children at different ages

It is intended that these tables are used only by professionals who work with children.

At the end of Chapters 1 to 4 are 'Key skills' tables that outline communication skills usually evident in children of different ages. All babies and children differ in their rates of development, including in their acquisition of communication skills. These tables, which are based on research, can be used as an overall guide of what to expect at different ages. They have not been standardized on any group of children. Speech and language therapists use a range of detailed, standardized tests to investigate children's language when indicated.

⚠ Tables outlining possible warning signs at different ages

Once again, these tables are intended for use only by professionals who work with children.

At the end of Chapters 1 to 4 are 'Warning sign' tables which contain suggestions of possible signs that a child is developing at a slower rate, for different ages. Sometimes communication skills do not develop as expected in babies and children. Although there are great differences among children regarding rates of development, it is best to address any parental or professional concerns that might arise. Any professional concern about a child's communication skills development must be discussed with parents before any action is taken. Any parental concern must be listened to and taken seriously. It is advisable to seek assessment of the child's communication skills by a speech and language therapist in circumstances described in the 'Possible warning signs' tables. Additional concerns regarding a child's development need to be discussed with parents and onward referrals for assessment made as appropriate.

Glossary

The glossary at the back of the book explains terms that may be unfamiliar to readers. Words in the glossary are marked the first time they appear in the book by the use of italics.

Belinda Buckley

Acknowledgements

I gratefully acknowledge the cooperation and contributions of all the children mentioned in this book, and of their caregivers. Thanks to my colleagues over the years, and to all who provided helpful comments on the book at its various stages. Special thanks to Barbara, Charlotte, Darryl and Rowan.

Acknowledgements to publishers

Thanks to the following, who generously granted permission for me to use materials from their publications as sources for tables in this book: Lippincott Williams & Wilkins, publishers of C.E. Westby (1998) 'Social-Emotional Bases of Communication Development', in W.O. Haynes and B.B. Shulman (eds) *Communication Development: Foundations, Processes and Clinical Applications*, Baltimore; Allyn & Bacon, Columbus; Cambridge University Press; Academic Press; Elsevier Press.

Introduction

Human communication

- What is meant by the terms *communication, language* and *speech*?
- How are communication, language and speech involved in expressing and understanding messages?
- Environmental and internal factors which contribute to the development of communication, language and speech.
- Summary of key points.

Communication, language and speech

Communication

What is communication?

The Chambers Dictionary (1998) defines the verb 'to communicate' as 'to succeed in conveying one's meaning to others.' Messages people send can be unintentional or *intentional*. For example, very young babies that have not yet learned about the purposes of communication nevertheless succeed in conveying messages to others through their cries and movements. Over the course of their development, children learn that communication is used to achieve different purposes (such as getting a drink, seeking comfort or telling a story). Children learn to become increasingly effective communicators as they succeed in both conveying and interpreting a wider range of messages and develop an understanding of how to respond appropriately. They learn that messages can be conveyed in different ways using different combinations of *nonverbal* and *verbal* means.

If communication is about conveying meaning (or 'messages') it necessarily involves:

- somebody who sends a message (for example a speaker, writer or signer)

- the message (which might be in the form of a wave, a prod, a laugh, a single *word* such as 'Hello' or a complete novel, for example)
- somebody who receives the message (for example by seeing it, hearing it or feeling it).

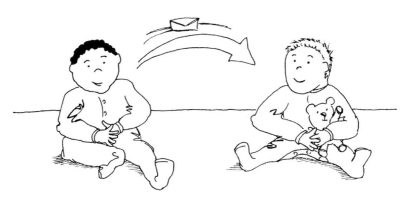

Figure I.1 The elements of communication: a message is sent by one person, and received by another

Why do humans communicate?

Humans are essentially social animals and communication skills are at the heart of social interaction. Developing communication skills enables children to exert control over their social and emotional worlds and to relate to others. The stages of communication skills development that children progress through provide the basis for successful communication in later life. Communication is fundamental to education and, as they move towards adulthood, people need communication skills in order to participate in all areas of life including work, leisure and relationships.

How do humans communicate?

Humans use both nonverbal and verbal channels to convey their meaning to others. Nonverbal communication includes eye gaze, facial expression, physical proximity, *gestures*, *vocalizations* and *body language*. Verbal communication refers to the use of language, which can be spoken or written. Messages can also be conveyed via other visual means such as symbols, pictures and *signs*. People receive *auditory* messages via their sense of hearing, visual messages via their sense of vision and *tactile* messages via their sense of touch. Most face-to-face interactions between humans involve a combination of nonverbal and verbal messages which might be visual, auditory and tactile. The person receiving the message must be able to integrate all the different incoming sensory information if the full meaning of the message is to be comprehended.

Language

What is language?

The definition of language has evolved over the course of the last century from one equating language with *grammar* (rules for combining words), to one that includes the contextual and functional aspects of communication. Mogford and Bishop (1993a) describe language as 'a system organized in a regular and predictable way such that it is possible to write a set of rules that describes the regularities of the system.' If the purpose of language is communication, then language is a rule-governed communication system. The system is composed of meaningful elements (sounds, words and signs for example) which can be combined according to rules to express an infinite range of meanings. The elements are arbitrary in that, particularly in spoken language, they bear no direct relationship to the things that they refer to. In this way, language is symbolic. This is one of the reasons why different languages have different words to refer to the same thing, for example 'hat' in English and 'châpeau' in French are used for the article of clothing worn on the head. *Onomatopoeic* words, such as 'tick-tock' for the sound of a ticking clock, exist in languages, however, and are one of the ways that young children break the language code, as they are easier to understand initially (Myers Pease *et al.* 1989). Once a rule-governed communication system is in operation among a group of speakers or signers (depending on whether the language is spoken or signed) then mutually intelligible communication is possible. Kamhi (1989) cites the definition endorsed by the American Speech-Language-Hearing Association (ASHA) in 1983:

> Language is a complex and dynamic system of conventional symbols that is used in various modes for thought and communication. Contemporary views of human language hold that: a) language evolves within specific historical, social, and cultural contexts; b) language, as rule-governed behaviour, is described by at least five parameters – phonologic, morphologic, syntactic, semantic, and pragmatic; c) language learning and use are determined by the interaction of biological, cognitive, psycho-social, and environmental factors; and d) effective use of language for communication requires a broad under-standing of human interaction including such associated factors as nonverbal cues, motivation, and socio-cultural roles.
>
> (Kamhi 1989: 69–70)

The evolution of language is beyond the scope of this book. An aim of this chapter is to raise the reader's awareness of the rule-governed and multi-levelled nature of language, and the role that language plays in the multi-layered process of human communication.

Language can be described, then, as being made up of the levels described below. (Grammar, which is to do with the internal structure of words and the structure of sentences, is used by some linguists, such as Mogford and Bishop 1993a, to refer to both *syntax* and morphology.)

- Phonology
  Phonology refers to how the sounds (*consonants* and *vowels*) that exist in a language are used *contrastively* to signal differences in meaning; different languages have different sound systems which are used in language-specific ways. English uses the sounds 'r' and 'l' contrastively which results in a difference in meaning between the words *rake* and *lake*. There is, however, no distinction between these two sounds in Japanese. This makes it hard for the Japanese learner of English to distinguish between 'r' and 'l' both perceptually and productively. Phonology also refers to how the sounds of the language may be organized and combined to form words. For example, the sound 'zh' as in 'measure' cannot occur at the beginning of English words, but can in French, e.g. 'je' (I), 'jour' (day). In English it is possible to combine the sounds 's' and 'p' at the start of words as in 'spy', but not 'k' and 'p' as in 'kpy'.

- Morphology
  Morphology refers to the group of words and *inflections* (*bound morphemes*) that exist in a language that subtly modify the meaning of a sentence, and the rules that govern their use. *Morphemes* are the smallest element of meaning in a language. In English there are *free morphemes* that stand alone (for example, 'cat') and bound morphemes that include the *plural* 's' as in cats ('the cats sleep by the fire' in contrast to 'the cat sleeps by the fire'), the *past tense* ending 'ed' to signal that an event took place in the past ('my dad cooked dinner', in contrast to 'my dad cooks dinner'). What differentiate the sentences in brackets are the grammatical morphemes, while the major elements of meaning are similar in the two pairs of sentences.

- Syntax
  Syntax refers to the rules that exist for combining different words into phrases and sentences so that they make sense. In English the sentence 'Dad cooks in the kitchen' makes sense but 'kitchen the Dad in cooks' does not. These rules specify the relationships between elements such as people, actions, things and their characteristics: 'who does what to whom'; 'whose is it?'; 'why did she do it?'; 'how did he do it?'; 'where is it?' and so on. In the sentence, 'Dad cooks in the kitchen' 'dad' is the subject of the verb 'cooks' and 'in the kitchen' refers to where the action took place, signalled by the position word 'in'. Different languages have different syntactic rules. Rules governing word order, for example, are far more flexible in Spanish than in English, where the same word order can be used to express both a question and a statement. For example, 'està en la cocina' could mean 'he is in the kitchen', or 'is he in the kitchen?' *Intonation* is used to specify the difference in meaning.

- Semantics
  Semantics refers to the meaning of words and of word combinations. The meaning of the word 'house' refers to its defining characteristics such as appearance and function (made of construction materials such as bricks, stones, wood; may be divided up inside into rooms; has an entrance such as a door;

has walls, floor and roof; may exist on more than one level; used for living in). The meaning of the phrase 'dad's house' depends on the relationship between the component words. Through combining these two words, the house is specified and the summative meaning is thus different from that of the phrase, 'grandma's house'.

- Pragmatics
Pragmatics refers to how language is used in context to serve a range of purposes. Pragmatics is constrained by sets of rules, like other levels of language. For example, there are rules about how to initiate, regulate and terminate *conversations*. Bates (1976) used the term 'pragmatics' to refer to:

  - how language and communication are used to communicate a range of meanings (for example requesting, persuading, informing)
  - how people adapt to the needs of a listener (a baby as opposed to a bank manager, for example) and
  - how people use language and communication to hold conversations.

It would be inappropriate for a teenager to start a conversation with his teacher by using the phrase, 'Oi, missus . . .'; the teenager's behaviour would be interpreted as rudeness, in most situations. Individuals can intentionally violate the rules of pragmatics in order to express rudeness or humour, for example; some individuals (including some diagnosed with autistic spectrum disorders) violate these rules without being aware that they do so, however.

Although it is possible to separate out the different levels of language in this way, it should be remembered that these levels do not develop in isolation in normal development but are interdependent. Development of the language, communication and speech systems are dependent on each other and inextricably interwoven into a child's general development. Children need to learn not only how to use language effectively but also to understand it when used by other people. Knowledge of the rules that exist in speech, language and communication is implicit in children acquiring the language and in mature speakers. Most English-speaking adults without linguistic training know instinctively that the combined words 'kitchen the dad in cooks' does not make sense, but would lack the explicit linguistic knowledge to state why this is so.

Why does language exist?

In addition to the communicative purposes of language already touched on, language is used to develop knowledge, for thinking, for reasoning and solving problems and for remembering. Language helps children learn about the world, allowing them to give names to things of interest and relevance and helping them to organize their knowledge of the world. New words represent new concepts learned, thus expanding knowledge about the world. Thus cats, monkeys, hamsters and cows come to be grouped together in the category referred to as 'animals' and buttons, balls, the sun and belly buttons are grouped together in the category of things that are 'round'. In addition to using language to refer to what exists in the here and now, it can be used to refer to things that are not immediately visible, about the future, the past and imaginary events. As language develops, it is used increasingly as a tool for thought and memory.

Speech

What is speech?

Speech involves the use of *speech sounds* to express language. Speech is only one form of expressing language – others are writing and *sign language*. Some people who never develop speech are able to read and write and some learn how to communicate using sign language, or other visual communication systems.

Speech can be considered as the sounds that result from a series of intricate muscular movements made in different parts of the mouth by a group of muscles (Figure I.2). The '*articulators*' are those parts of the mouth and muscles involved in producing speech: lips, tongue, *soft palate* (soft muscular flap at the back of the mouth which is open for breathing and usually closes off the nasal cavity for speech), roof of mouth, *pharynx* (throat) and jaw. In mature speech, the articulators move in automatic and specific ways according to learned patterns of *pronunciations* for words that are stored in the mind (Hewlett 1990, Crary 1993, Stackhouse and Wells 1997). Each word that a mature speaker utters has its own *articulatory pattern*; one aspect of speech development in children is the development of such mental patterns of word pronunciation which is necessary for automatic and error-free speech. Establishment of these patterns is partially informed by the child's *perception* of words that are spoken by others. This is why children grow up speaking the *accent* used by speakers they interact with when learning to speak. It is necessary, then, to establish reliable auditory perceptual patterns for words in order to achieve accurate pronunciations. Children need to be able to perceive the difference in how pairs of words such as *boy* and *bee*, *boy* and *toy* sound before they can signal the difference in their pronunciation of these words. There is further discussion of the development of speech in the relevant sections of Chapters 1 to 4.

How is speech produced?

Speech involves extremely fast, coordinated sequences of muscular movements that take place in the *vocal tract* (Borden and Harris 1984). The vocal tract is a name given to the air passages involved in speech production and extends from the *larynx* upwards to include the throat and mouth cavities and the nasal cavity (Figure I.3). A sequence of the basic muscular movements that occur when producing the word 'boy' appears below:

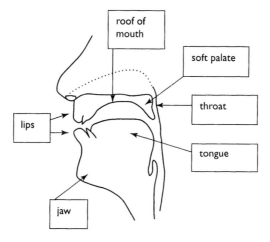

Figure 1.2 The physical structures involved in articulating speech – the articulators

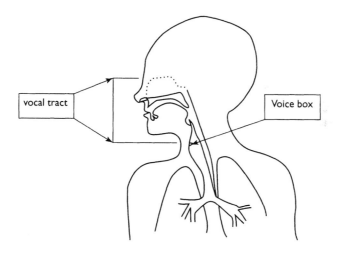

Figure 1.3 The vocal tract (the air passages above the larynx)

- diaphragm and ribcage muscles relax and air is exhaled from the lungs
- lips meet as soft palate closes off the nose from the throat – air builds up inside the mouth
- exhaled air is released from the mouth as the lips part and the *vocal folds* in the *voice box* start vibrating ('b' is uttered)

- the bottom jaw lowers and the bunched up tongue moves downwards and forwards as the vocal folds continue to vibrate ('oy' is uttered).

Part of the reason why normal speech sounds fluent is because it is produced with precision timing and a high level of coordination between *articulations* of sounds (Borden and Harris 1984). Thus the sounds 'b' + 'oy' (boy) are uttered in smooth, coordinated sequence.

Speech is made on exhaled air from the lungs (it can be made on inspiration, though is not as effective), entailing coordination of respiratory function and speech production. When exhaled air passes through the vibrating vocal folds in the voice box, *voice* is the result. The throat, mouth, nasal cavity and sinuses around the nose act as resonating chambers that give the voice its human and individual quality. However, other muscle movements are necessary to convert the sound of voice into recognizable speech. Recognizable speech is the result of a series of speech sounds (consonants and vowels) being produced in a particular sequence which match the listener's auditory perceptual pattern of the word being uttered. Some speech sounds in English such as 's', 'k', and 'f' are made on exhaled air but without activation of the vocal folds. In order to say the word 'far' in a recognizable way, the speaker has to coordinate activation of the vocal folds at the right time – at the transition between the production of 'f' and that of the vowel sound. The sounds 'z', 'g' and 'v' are made in the same place in the mouth, and in the same way as the previous three sounds mentioned. The difference is that these three are made with vibration of the vocal folds in the voice box (also called 'voicing').

Another way of illustrating the highly intricate, complex and precise nature of muscular movements involved in speech is to consider the sound of an unknown foreign language being spoken (Borden and Harris 1984). The spoken language sounds like long spurts of a complex and constantly changing stream of sound without separations. It is extremely difficult, without knowing a language, to identify the beginnings and ends of words. It might appear that speakers of the foreign language speak much more quickly than speakers of one's own language. These impressions are more precisely descriptions of speech itself. Speakers take their own speech for granted. However, it is the most complicated *motor* task facing young children, involving thirty-six different muscles (Borden and Harris 1984).

Additional information to the meaning that is conveyed on coded speech sounds is carried in the voice itself. Voices tell listeners about the emotional state of the speaker – loud voices signal anger; trembling voices suggest shock, fear or anxiety; flat voices might indicate depression. The way the voice is used in combination with the actual words spoken informs the listener of the type of message conveyed – whether the words 'I'm sorry' signal an apology, a request for repetition or an expression of disdain, for example. This type of information is signalled by changes of loudness, changes of pitch and temporal features such as pauses and rate of speech.

The multi-factorial nature of human communication

What factors are involved in communication?

The following factors play a role in human communication:

- the motivation to engage in communication
- the situation in which the communication takes places (the office at work, the bathroom at home, the nursery play area, the doctor's surgery, a grandmother's dinner table)
- the relationship between the participants and their roles relative to each other (work colleagues, husband and wife, teacher and pupil, doctor and patient, grandmother and grandchild)
- the type of message that is conveyed (a request for information, a comment, an instruction, an answer, a request for an object)
- the ability to *take turns* as both speaker and listener
- the ability to comprehend and use nonverbal messages
- the ability to comprehend and use verbal messages
- the ability to modify messages produced as a result of *feedback* from the listener, and of feedback provided by one's own body (*auditory feedback* of one's own speech for example).

If an individual is not motivated to communicate, there will be no communication, or it will be limited. This – the desire not to communicate with others – might be considered a form of communication in itself in some circumstances. Situations, relationships and roles of speakers determine what type of communication takes place – it is to be expected that a nursery teacher will give children lots of instructions, but it would not be thought appropriate for the children to instruct the teachers in the same manner. Likewise, it is acceptable and within expectations that a doctor will ask a patient about her symptoms, but not appropriate for the patient to inquire of the doctor's. The type of message that is conveyed in any communicative situation is determined again partly by the situation in terms of what is appropriate and what conforms to one's expectations of that situation, and partly by what type of message the speakers intend to convey. Violations of expectations regarding social interaction and communication in given situations might be intentional or not (see page 5).

Individuals need to develop the ability to both receive messages (by looking and *listening*) and convey messages, in order to comprehend other people and express themselves effectively, both of which are necessary to two-way communication. Individuals need to be able to hear, see, process and comprehend incoming verbal and visual information for optimal comprehension of the other person's message. They need to want to do this, as they need to want to express themselves in some way to the other person, in order for communication to take place. In order to express themselves, they need to have something to communicate about, to be able to formulate the message through language and nonverbal means and then execute that message using coordinated speech and gesture, for example. They need to be able to identify when communication has broken down and why, and attempt to *repair* it through modifying their message or requesting clarification, depending on whether they are the listener or the speaker.

This section has so far dealt with key motivational, situational, and communication factors in sending and receiving messages. It is necessary also to look at the *mental processing* involved in comprehending and producing speech for both speaker and listener for a fuller appreciation of the multi-factorial nature of human communication. Figures I.4 and I.5 schematize these processes. Gross (1992) defines mental processes as 'those ways in which knowledge of the world is attained, retained and used'. Processes such as those central to *verbal understanding* and speech production can only be inferred and not seen directly. It is necessary to point out that there is no real time equivalent suggested for any aspect of mental processing; processing of the different types of information is thought to occur in a parallel, rather than serial manner (Garman 1990).

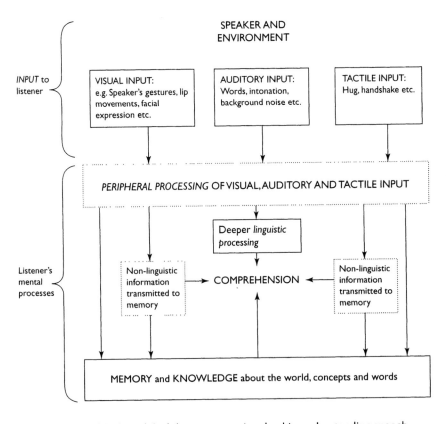

Figure *I.4* A simplified model of the processes involved in understanding speech
Source: Adapted from Garman 1990 with the permission of Cambridge University Press.

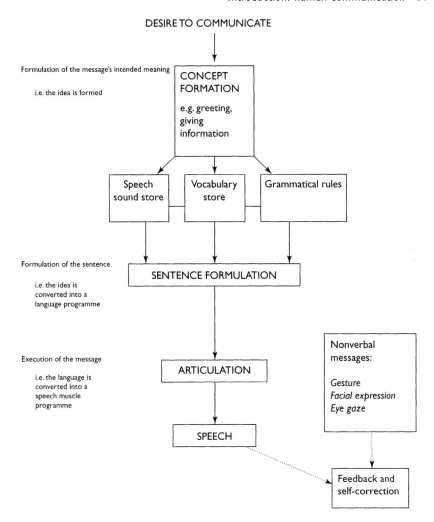

DESIRE TO COMMUNICATE

Formulation of the message's intended meaning

i.e. the idea is formed

CONCEPT
FORMATION

e.g. greeting,
giving
information

Speech
sound store

Vocabulary
store

Grammatical rules

Formulation of the sentence

i.e. the idea is
converted into a
language programme

SENTENCE FORMULATION

Execution of the message

i.e. the language is
converted into a
speech muscle
programme

ARTICULATION

Nonverbal
messages:

*Gesture
Facial expression
Eye gaze*

SPEECH

Feedback and
self-correction

Figure 1.5 A simplified model of the processes involved in producing speech
Source: Garman 1990.

Understanding speech

The factors involved at each of the stages in understanding speech as illustrated
in Figure I.4, are expanded on here. Understanding speech involves more than
comprehending the speech signal alone: other available information, in the form of
simultaneous and preceding visual information (for example nonverbal communication, preceding messages exchanged in the interaction, the knowledge stored
in memory for words and situations, and the expectations the listener has of the
interaction), impinges on comprehension of speech (Garman 1990). A summary of
the factors necessary for comprehension of speech follows:

- The listener needs to be able to hear the *acoustic* signal.
- The listener needs to be able to attend to a new signal and treat it as salient information.
- The listener needs to have intact *auditory processing*. This involves analysis of the sounds of incoming speech and is a precursor to comprehending speech. For example, listeners are able to hear a foreign language spoken and might be able to identify which language it is (recognition of speech) but will not necessarily be able to understand the meaning.
- There needs to be integration of speech *input* with other incoming information (visual and situational factors). This is necessary for full comprehension of the spoken message. *Peripheral processing*, i.e. initial processing of incoming auditory, visual and other forms of sensory input, is integrated among the senses and does not involve comprehension.
- There needs to be transmission of the auditory information that has undergone auditory processing for further *linguistic processing* (for example, application of knowledge about grammatical rules and word meanings which assist in the process of comprehension).
- The listener needs to have words, concepts and knowledge in their memory that will enable them to make sense of the incoming information.
- The listener uses their knowledge of the speaker and the situation to inform their comprehension of the message.
- The listener uses information from visual, tactile and other sources to inform their comprehension of the message.
- The listener integrates all relevant information to arrive at comprehension of the message.

Deficits in any of these areas can result in a *receptive* communication problem. In reference to the processes involved in comprehending *utterances*, Garman (1990) points out that '*understanding* . . . is not a place to be reached, or a set of processes, but the result of a number of interactions, in dynamic balance.'

Producing speech

The factors involved in producing speech as shown in Figure I.5 are expanded upon here. Producing meaningful speech, or any form of meaningful message, starts with having something to communicate about. The intended meanings of messages are concepts that can be coded into language and expressed through speech, for example. Once an intended meaning (such as a greeting) has been formulated conceptually by a speaker, the underlying concept or concepts are 'mapped onto' the language code (Garman 1990). This involves accessing words from an individual's mental *vocabulary store* and speech sounds from their *speech sound store*, and applying grammatical rules that comprise part of the speaker's implicit knowledge about their language. A sentence is consequently formulated and, in the case of speech, messages are sent from the brain to the articulators and the utterance is articulated. Auditory feedback (of the utterance produced) and *visual feedback* (listener's facial expression and movements, for example) provide the speaker with information regarding the effectiveness and accuracy of their utterance. *Proprioceptive* feedback, which is to do with knowing where in the body the articulators and other muscles are positioned, is another important source of information to the speaker about the effectiveness and accuracy of their utterance. One way to illustrate this is to think about what it feels like to talk immediately after a visit to the dentist, having experienced an oral anaesthetic. One effect of the anaesthetic is to disturb oral proprioception, thus affecting knowledge that a person has about where in the mouth their tongue is positioned, for example. Without accurate information of this type, articulation is imprecise, which can impact on the intelligibility of the utterance. A summary of the factors necessary to producing meaningful speech follows:

- The speaker needs to have intact memory, conceptual, language and *speech processing* capabilities.
- The speaker needs to have something to say (an intended meaning).
- The speaker needs to have an *expressive vocabulary* containing words that can express the intended meaning.
- The speaker needs to know how to use grammar (put words in the right order and with the right word endings) to specify the intended meaning.
- The speaker needs to know how to use speech sounds accurately.
- The speaker needs to have intact structure and functioning of articulators.
- The speaker needs to be able to coordinate nonverbal and verbal channels of communication.
- The speaker needs to have intact hearing and vision so he can receive feedback of his message.

Deficits in any of these areas can result in an expressive communication difficulty.

An exchange of messages

In the following example an exchange of messages takes place between a 4-year-old boy, Jake, and his father. The key motivational, situational, communication, language, speech, *attention* and sensory factors involved at each stage of the exchange are specified.

1   Jake is sitting at home in the early evening watching television in the sitting room. His mother is in the kitchen preparing dinner.

Factors:
- Jake has intact hearing and vision.
- Jake attends to the visual and auditory information from the television.
- Jake usually watches television at this time of day.

2   Jake's father arrives home at the usual time. He looks in to the sitting room and sees that Jake is watching the television. Jake is facing away from the sitting room door, so his father can only see the back of his head.

Factors:
- Jake's father usually arrives home at this time of day.
- Jake's father 'reads the situation'.
- Jake's father has intact hearing and vision.

3   Jake's father says, 'Hello Jake, I'm home!'

Factors:
- Jake's father is pleased to see his son.
- He wants to greet Jake and let him know that he is home (intended meaning).
- His brain maps the intended meaning of the message on to the language code.
- His brain sends messages to his articulators (lips, tongue, etc.) to articulate the message.
- He speaks, using words that convey his intended meaning – 'Hello Jake, I'm home!', thus initiating interaction with Jake.
- He receives auditory feedback of his own speech, which confirms that the spoken message that he has uttered is correct and matches his intended meaning.

4   Jake turns his head towards his father in the doorway and responds by smiling, getting up, running towards him, hugging him, kissing him and saying 'Daddy!'

Factors:
- Jake hears his father's spoken message.
- Jake attends to the spoken message, treating it as salient (new) auditory information.
- Jake processes the auditory information.
- Jake uses the *nonlinguistic* information from the situation to inform his comprehension (he was anticipating seeing his father as he had heard the car draw up outside, he was expecting his father home at this time, his father usually greets him from the doorway when he is watching television).
- Jake understands the meaning of his father's utterance, and that it is directed at him.
- Jake turns his head away from the television and towards his father – now that he is in the same room he is more interested in him than the television programme.
- Jake is pleased that his father is home.
- Jake wants to express delight at seeing his father by greeting him.
- Jake and his father make eye contact and smile at each other.
- Jake gets up from the floor and runs towards his father.
- Jake's father opens his arms in anticipation of a hug.

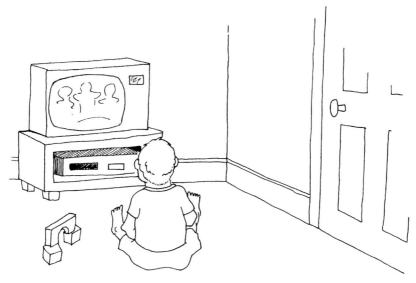

Figure I.6 Jake watching television

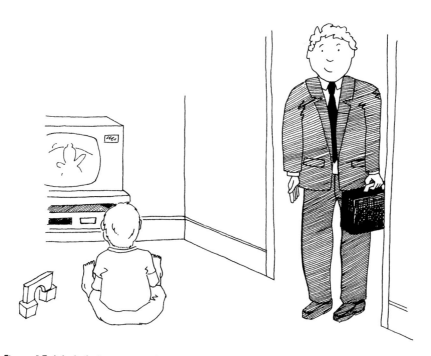

Figure I.7 Jake's father arrives home

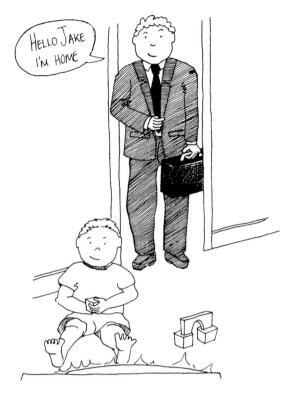

Figure I.8 Jake is greeted by his father

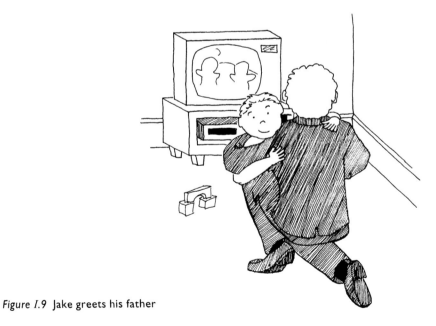

Figure I.9 Jake greets his father

- Jake and his father make close physical contact by hugging.
- Jake speaks, using a word that conveys his intended meaning (greeting) 'Daddy!'
- Jake's father receives auditory, visual and tactile feedback that confirm that his message has been comprehended.
- Jake receives visual and tactile feedback that confirm that his message has been comprehended.

What do children need to develop communication, language and speech?

Having looked at the key components of human communication and discussed its multi-factorial nature, it is now possible to consider what children need in order to develop their communication skills. A subtle combination and interaction of environmental and internal factors contribute to the development of speech, language and communication in children. A summary of these factors is presented below and expanded on in the relevant sections of the following chapters. It is important to point out that individuals differ significantly regarding the interaction of these factors and how they impinge on speech, language and communication development (Lees and Urwin 1991). Circumstances in which children develop differ vastly, too. There is no hard and fast 'recipe' of factors and influences for optimal communication development in children, but a minimum threshold in each general area is necessary for normal development of communication skills. Childhood communication difficulties form the content of Chapter 6 and links are drawn between the factors involved in speech, language and communication, the prerequisites for development of these in children and the types of difficulties that arise. Figure 6.1 (page 181) schematizes internal and environmental factors which impact on communication skills development.

Internal factors

- Children need to want to communicate.
- Children need to have social interest, social awareness and knowledge about social interaction.
- Children need to know what communication is for.
- Children need intact senses (especially hearing and vision).
- Children need intact *neurological* growth and development.
- Children need intact structural growth and development, for example of the *respiratory system*, voice box and articulators.
- Children need to have intact cognitive development.
- Children need to have intact *perceptual* and *mental processing* capabilities for speech, language and learning.

Environmental factors

- Children need secure, affectionate relationships with caregivers which motivate them to communicate and which provide feedback on their communication.
- Children need interaction opportunities with familiar and unfamiliar adults and peers to learn about cultural and social conventions and appropriate social interaction, and to support the development of their communication skills (initiating, responding, greeting, requesting, protesting, taking turns, for example) in different contexts (at home, at nursery, at a party, in museums and cinemas, for example).
- Children need opportunities for interaction with adults in order to hear spoken language and develop their understanding of it, and in order to use their developing *expressive language*.
- Children benefit from hearing language addressed to them which is in tune with their current level of understanding. For younger children this includes a smaller, simplified *vocabulary*, grammatically simple phrases and sentences, exaggerated pitch and exaggerated pronunciation of key words.
- Children need to experience events which provide opportunities for learning associated concepts and language. Frequently repeated routines such as having a bath and getting dressed enable children to consolidate and reinforce their learning of the situation and related language. As children get older, non-routine events become increasingly important for learning and using less familiar language.
- Children need to learn about the world through experiencing it, especially through play. They need access to a wide range of play opportunities and things in the world (animals, books, toys, everyday objects) to support all areas of development including cognition, language and social understanding.

Further environmental influences

Dialects and accents

All languages consist of a range of *dialects* (referring to grammar, idiom and vocabulary) and accents (referring to pronunciation). The notion that there is one and only one correct form of a language (a 'standard language ideology') has been the topic of media attention and public interest over the years. There is no dialect which is, however, as a *linguistic* system, any better in terms of logic or effectiveness than another (Labov 1972, Trudgill 1975, Edwards 1979).

In the United Kingdom, Standard English is the dialect which, for historical and social reasons, has high levels of social prestige (Labov 1972, Trudgill 1975, Edwards 1979). Proposals to teach spoken Standard English to all children in British schools were put forward in the Cox Report (Department of Education and Science 1988) so that 'Children should be able to communicate not only with families and the local community, but also in the wider community and in public life' (Paragraph

4.24). The Cox Report claims that many areas of further and higher education, cultural, industrial, commercial areas and the professions are largely closed to non-Standard English-speakers.

Milroy (2001) reports how sociolinguists in the United Kingdom have attempted to counter linguistic discrimination in the classroom by stressing the linguistic equality of all dialects and recommending tolerance of a child's home accent or dialect. This is especially true when children are being taught to read and write in a dialect other than their own.

Although no dialect is capable of greater expression than another (Trudgill 1975), different dialects contain more elaborated vocabularies than others, reflecting their particular uses. For example, Standard English vocabulary is more elaborated in some areas than non-Standard English dialects because of its uses in academic and administrative areas. Similarly, each non-Standard dialect has the potential for such elaboration, and certain non-Standard dialects' vocabularies are more elaborated than others, depending on speakers' needs. A related discussion pertaining to *bilingualism* can be found on pages 154–157.

The British educational sociolinguist Basil Bernstein (1975) characterized two key styles of speech among speakers of English, which he referred to as 'elaborated code' and 'restricted code'. Elaborated code contains more unusual words, passives ('the bone was gnawed by the dog' instead of 'the dog gnawed the bone'), modals (should, ought, would) and proliferation of subjective phrases such as 'I think', 'In my opinion', 'Personally'. Bernstein identified elaborated code as a style of speech used by many (middle and upper class) Standard English speakers. Labov (1972) drew a contrast between speakers who use elaborated code and who appear knowledgeable while not dealing precisely with abstract ideas, and the more effective narrative, reasoning and debating skills illustrated by users of restricted code. This style of speaking involves a more direct style of expression, using the immediate context to express meanings. The restricted code was identified by Bernstein as a style of speech characteristic of working classes in the United Kingdom.

The role of the linguistic environment in early language development

Related to Bernstein's restricted and elaborated codes is the question of the role of the linguistic environment in children's language development. In a most basic form, linguistic input functions as the language model which most children eventually achieve, in that most grow up speaking the language of their environment. Input is thus clearly necessary. Two key questions have arisen concerning how language input might influence children's language acquisition:

- Does the language that children hear act merely as a trigger, catalyzing children's predisposition to learn language and through this assist them in working out the rules of their language (such as the need in English to invert the subject

and *verb* in order to transform a statement into a question, for example 'John likes blue shoes' → 'Does John like blue shoes?'); and if so, to what extent?
- Do the special features present in so much speech directed to babies and young children serve to facilitate language development, and if so, how?

Many adults and older children (especially from western cultures) use simplifying, clarifying and affective features in speech addressed to babies and young children, distinguishing it from adult-to-adult speech. This form of speech, or register, has variously been termed '*motherese*' (Newport 1976) and '*child directed talk*' (Warren-Leubecker and Bohannon III 1989). The 'Motherese Hypothesis' resulted from research looking at the effect of adult (usually maternal) speech on language development. Ferguson (1977) claimed that many simplifying processes in motherese assisted in teaching language, which she maintained was the primary function of the register. Such processes include a smaller, simplified vocabulary, a rudimentary grammar with restricted, structurally simple sentence types, and fewer sound types and combinations of words. Ferguson noted that simplified language is accelerated in terms of complexity as the child's language progresses, drawing the conclusion that a cause and effect relationship existed between such features and language development. Garnica (1977) concluded that exaggerated use of features such as *vocal* pitch, pausing and longer duration of some words in motherese assisted children in deriving grammatical information about the language.

It is plausible that special features of this register have some function with regard to language learning, but opinion is divided concerning the degree to which functions are based in 'teaching' language and enabling communication.

A major tenet of the Motherese Hypothesis, that 'restrictive sentences' (i.e. in structure) are a requirement for language learning, has been challenged by Gleitman *et al.* (1984).

Against this background of claims and challenges regarding the role of adult speech in facilitating children's language development, the following research findings are worthy of note:

- A shared focus of attention between the baby or young child and the adult, which is a basic principle of shared communication, increases the likelihood of early vocabulary growth (Tomasello and Ferrar 1986, Garton 1992).
- An extended pitch range, including whispering and high pitch especially, particularly at the end of adult utterances, cues the child as to when she's expected to respond. This, together with frequent repetitions of the child's name, serves to establish and maintain the child's attention (Garnica 1977).
- Children exploit some of the linguistic input some of the time (Gleitman *et al.* 1984); i.e. children make use of the language they hear in different ways at different points of their development, and depending on their stage of language development at that time.
- 'Simple' input may be more facilitative for younger (18- to 21-month-old) children's task of learning vocabulary and producing simple phrases for a basic range of purposes, whereas more complex input may be required for older (24-

to 27-month-old) children's task of acquiring word endings and grammatical rules (Snow 1986).

- The restricted range of vocabulary spoken by mothers to young children, focusing on words with the simplest and most unambiguous meanings, for example kin, the body, qualities, animals, games and food, constituting the here and now, enables children to figure out the meanings of words (Ferguson 1977).
- Adults' ability to match and anticipate a child's cognitive level is observed at the level of word meanings (semantic fine tuning), which benefits semantic development (Myers Pease *et al.* 1989). For example, an adult might label both lorries and cars as 'car' for a child at an early stage of language development. Later on, they might label them in such a way as to facilitate understanding of the relations that exist between word meanings and the entities they represent, for example 'lorries, cars, buses . . . they've all got wheels!'
- A positive relation was identified between gradually increasing complexity of language spoken to children and children's language growth (Gleitman *et al.* 1984).
- Better formed sentences by young children result from adults requesting clarification rather than making grammatical corrections (Garton 1992).
- Parents tend to correct the factual accuracy of children's language rather than how it is said (Snow 1986).
- Children of mothers whose language contained many commands designed to control their behaviour were described by Folger and Chapman (1977) as being 'more inclined to act than talk', and their vocabulary contained a greater number of personal and social words (for example, hello, bye, yeah, no, mine) than descriptive words (for example, big, more, wet, sticky).
- Children of mothers whose language contained more descriptions of the environment and requests for information had a greater number of object names in their vocabulary (Della-Corte *et al.* 1983).

Further information on ways in which adults adapt their communication, and babies' response to this, appears on pages 32–33. It is not only adults, however, who adapt their communication to match the needs of the listener; children as young as 4 were found to use more attention-getting and attention-holding words with 2-year-olds than with adults (Hetherington and Parke 1986).

Summary of introduction

Communication, language and speech

1 The basic elements of human communication are a person who expresses a message, the message itself and the person who receives the message.
2 Most human communication involves a combination of nonverbal and verbal messages that might be auditory, visual and tactile.

3 Language is a symbolic, rule-governed communication system composed of meaningful elements that can be combined in an infinite variety of ways to achieve a vast range of purposes in any context.

4 A language can be described and analysed in terms of its phonology, morphology, syntax, semantics and pragmatics.

5 Knowledge that individuals develop about speech, language and communication is mostly implicit.

6 Language is used to assist communication, learning, thinking and remembering.

7 Speech is the acoustic signal resulting from a series of intricate and complex movements made by the articulators and is one way of expressing language, in addition to visual forms of communication such as signing.

8 Auditory perceptual processes are as important for the development of speech as productive processes.

9 Speech production is the most intricate, complex and precise motor skill humans ever have to learn.

The multi-factorial nature of human communication

10 Human communication is multi-factorial and involves factors related to motivation, the situation, attention and listening, sensory and motor functioning, comprehension of verbal and nonverbal messages and production of verbal and nonverbal messages.

What do children need to develop communication, language and speech?

11 A subtle interaction and combination of environmental and internal factors contribute to the development of speech, language and communication in children.

Further environmental influences

12 A language may have several dialects and accents; although no dialect or accent carries any linguistic superiority, it can carry social prestige.

13 Adaptations of adult speech have been observed to assist some children in acquiring language and to enable communication at different points of their development. These observations have been made of speakers in western societies.

The first year   1

Hearing, attention and listening

'Wired up' to hear voices

Babies are highly sensitive and attuned to the sounds of the human voice. Many babies quiet to the sound of a familiar, friendly voice from the earliest days after birth (Ashmead and Lipsitt 1977). The voice that they are most used to hearing is that of their mother. At twenty weeks, an embryo's inner ear (the part of the ear that senses and directs sounds on to the brain) is fully developed, which means that by the time a full-term baby is born, she has been hearing for about five months (Northern and Downs 1991). Babies only a few days old have shown preference for hearing their mother's voice over other voices and they are able to discriminate their mother's voice from other female voices (De Casper and Fifer 1980). Studies have also shown that newborn babies respond to and prefer the human voice over other sounds (Friedlander 1970). Other studies have shown that newborns respond to sound in different ways, depending on the duration, loudness and pitch of the sound. Newborn infants are predisposed, it would appear, to listen to the human voice and also to begin the mammoth task of separating out the various speech sounds from the streams of singing and speaking that envelope them from their earliest moments.

Development of hearing, attention and listening over the first year

The first six months: Developing selectivity

At birth, babies show a *startle response* to sudden changes in their environment. They may blink their eyes open wide or wake up from sleeping in response to loud noises, bright lights and sudden movement (Northern and Downs 1991). Their ability to control their attention is extremely limited in the first few weeks, enabling them to look at toys or faces for a very short space of time. Over the next few weeks, babies appear to listen to people speaking to them by looking and smiling at them (Bzoch and League 1991). They begin to show interest in speakers' mouths and by the end of the third month may start to look in the direction in which another person is looking. They quiet when they hear their parent's voice, even if the parent is not in view, and by 4 months babies will deliberately turn their heads towards the source of the voice, looking about for the speaker (Bzoch and League 1991). By 6 months the baby is still very distractible, but she is starting to become more selective towards sound. She will soon turn her head immediately to her parent's voice or to quieter sounds at the side of her head providing she is not preoccupied with a toy. She may show that she recognizes frequently heard names and words that are meaningful to her like 'mummy', 'daddy' and 'bye-bye' and may show early understanding of 'no' by stopping or hesitating in an activity (Bzoch and League 1991). The baby at this stage is only able to attend to input from one sensory channel at a time; when exploring a toy with her hands or watching an exciting mobile her lack of responsiveness to sound, for example, may make her appear deaf. The baby is getting better at being able to look in the same direction in which another person is looking and is beginning to share *joint attention* with another person towards an object or activity. Sharing joint attention is an extremely important skill to develop as it underpins later language and discourse skills.

The second six months: Listening to speech

Over the next five months the baby will come to recognize words in speech-action games, and start to attend to music and singing (Bzoch and League 1991). She will engage in sound-making activities such as banging spoons, pots and toys together. By now she can hold objects in either hand and bring her hands together (Sheridan 1997). She enjoys playing with squeaky toys and starts to respond to *representational sounds* such as animal and machine noises (moo, baabaa, vroom, brrrrroooom). By 8 months she may appear to listen to conversations between other people and to recognize the names of some everyday objects, and now regularly stops an activity when she hears 'no' (Bzoch and League 1991). Her attention span remains very limited, as is her ability to attend to information from more than one sense at a time. By this time she is able to follow an adult's pointing finger and to follow another person's gaze without difficulty, both of which contribute significantly to the amount of shared focus held between baby and adult (Carpenter *et al.* 1998). This mutual focus both helps the baby to understand the world around her and begin to see it from another person's perspective, and informs adults of what the baby is interested in. This last point is extremely important in enabling the baby to build up links between words and their meanings, which she is increasingly able to do in the forthcoming months. Around 10 months she is usually able to listen to other people talking and not be distracted by other sounds, and will often give a toy or some other object to a parent when asked to (Bzoch and League 1991). She can attend to an activity or object of her own choosing for a limited time. She is beginning to attend to visual and auditory information simultaneously for short periods of time. She may respond to music by moving her body or hand in approximate time to the rhythm. By the time she is a year old she will show intense attention and response to speech over prolonged periods of time. She is less distractible and is better able to look and listen at the same time. The ability to locate accurately sounds to the side, above and below ear level continues to develop and may not be fully developed until she is about 16 months old (Northern and Downs 1991).

Towards early verbal understanding

Cognitive developments

Developing concepts of objects

Babies need to know that objects like teddies, cups and blankets exist even when they are not in sight in order to give them names and talk about them when they are not there. The concept of *object permanence* starts developing around 5 months and may not be fully developed until the second year (Bloom 1993). Children's ability to represent objects, people and events mentally is closely linked to language development and other ways of symbolic representation of things in the world, especially play. The slightly older child can think about her favourite food, ask for it when it is not there and talk about it in conversation; later on she can turn a piece of cardboard or a wooden brick into a piece of cake in her play. Symbolic understanding is a very important part of learning to use language effectively. Once babies come to realize that things and people still exist even if they can't be seen and that actions can be remembered and anticipated ('Where did mummy put my teddy? I bet I'll find him in here!') they will have cause to use language to express their comments and discoveries to people they are interested in. Before they can start to use language effectively, however, babies need to understand language, and in order to do that they need to have plenty of experience of the things in the world that are represented by language (Bloom and Lahey 1978).

Objects and categories

Information gained through experiences about the perceptual and functional properties of objects enables the baby to start forming categories and thus to start linking labels not only to objects but also to their various features. Formation of conceptual categories, which are necessary in order for meaningful language to emerge (Bloom 1993) are built on the baby's concepts of objects. For example, the baby comes to understand that big and little spoons, plastic, metal and wooden spoons, pretend and real-life spoons can all be used for the same purpose – feeding. The baby needs to develop such categorical and conceptual information before she can start talking about big spoons or little spoons, or to differentiate spoons from forks, for example. Groupings of categories are very broad initially and become increasingly specified as the baby acquires more knowledge about things in the world around her (Mandler *et al.* 1991).

Example 1.1 Using objects in early play

At 10 months, Rowan started to put a brush briefly to her hair, to lift up and aim the television and video controls towards the television, to 'talk' into the telephone and to 'eat' from a spoon while she was at play. In these ways she demonstrated understanding of an object's use or meaning by using it, if only with a brief gesture, outside the normal context.

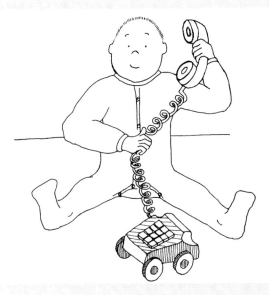

Figure 1.1 Ten-month-old Rowan uses a telephone in play

Early situational understanding

Between 6 and 12 months, babies' verbal understanding starts to develop. Babies gradually start to make associations between caregivers' words and gestures in familiar situations and routines such as feeding or changing. For example, a 9- to 10-month-old baby will give a toy she is holding to her father when she hears the words 'give to daddy' and sees her mother pointing in her father's direction. She will clap her hands when she hears the words 'clap hands' and sees her mother clapping her hands. At 12 months she will fetch a familiar object such as a beaker from the usual place on hearing, 'Where's your beaker?' in a routine situation such as feeding. She will point to body parts such as 'tummy', 'feet' and 'nose' when they are named and will point to named pictures in familiar books. She will show understanding of simple phrases like 'breakfast', 'daddy's here', 'your shoes' and a range of very familiar vocabulary.

Learning through experience and play

Through everyday activities and play, babies come to learn about objects in their world. They learn about the uses and appearance of objects, and about similarities and differences between them (Bloom 1993). Babies find out about relationships between people and objects, and learn through their own observations and experiences about the various effects of these. For example, the baby comes to learn the shape and feel of a ball; she observes how it is thrown up in the air, and how it then falls downwards, bounces on the ground and goes up in the air again. She sees how it rolls across the floor, and comes to learn that it will only do this if somebody sets it in motion. The baby will perceive a similarity between an orange and a ball (both are round and can roll on the floor). However, oranges do not bounce; they are for eating and they have tough skins that need peeling in order to get to the juicy bits inside. The baby's experience of playing with a ball, playing with an orange, eating an orange and putting a ball to her mouth will help to teach her about the various properties of these two objects, and help her understand about their different uses and thus why other people act on them in different ways.

Play and everyday experience with different objects help babies to learn about general effects of movement such as disappearance, reappearance and relocation of objects. Early conceptual development precedes, and is closely linked to, emergence of early words such as 'up', 'down', 'out', 'more', 'gone'. Similarly, babies come to learn that certain types of objects move (balls, dogs and cars) and others do not (houses, walls, lawns) – this knowledge is closely reflected in early vocabulary, which more typically consists of names of objects that potentially move (Bloom 1993). The baby more readily learns words that relate to actions that have specific effects on herself (eat, drink, fall down) including those actions performed by somebody else (swing, tickle).

Communication and expressive skills in the first year: why do babies communicate?

Preintentional and intentional communication

Until recently in the field of developmental psychology, a clear distinction has been drawn between '*preintentional*' and 'intentional' *communication* (Bruner 1973, Bates *et al.* 1975, Bates 1979). Communication in the preintentional infant (0 to 9 months) was essentially considered to be *reflexive*, occurring in response to internal or external stimuli, in contrast to intentional communication – occurring due to the child's intention to bring about some change or effect some response from people in the environment. Where the content of the younger baby's interactions with a caregiver refers only to herself and her caregiver, the older baby is able to indicate, through increasingly conventional use of eye gaze and gesture possibly combined with vocalizations or words, her desire for objects and also to direct another person's attention to an interesting object or event. During the second half of the first year, the baby starts to involve a third party (a toy, for example) in the interaction between herself and her caregiver. However, Reddy questions whether preintentional communication is qualitatively different from intentional communication. She notes that:

> while language may have a special place in sharing the contents of the mind, it is clearly not a unique place. Nonverbal actions already embody and reveal not only emotional states, intentions, interests, and thoughts (e.g. surprise or puzzlement) but also their targets.
>
> (Reddy 1999: 32)

Reddy argues that it is false to take the position that younger babies do not have communicative intent: communication needs to be considered as a two-way process between the baby and caregiver. She describes how young babies and caregivers actively engage in mutually pleasurable and balanced interactions. Reddy argues for an understanding of early infant communication based on the perspective that it is the 'continual elaboration of actions and intentions in response to the other's actions'.

Motivation to communicate

In order to start making sense of words and sentences, young language learners need to make attempts to crack the code for themselves. An essential prerequisite, therefore, is the desire to communicate with others. Bates *et al.* (in press) state that this motivation underlies the many hours undertaken by babies and children in 'attending, imitating, practising and contemplating the linguistic input'.

Caregiver as interpreter

The context in which communication takes place between babies and caregivers provides crucial information and cues that assist caregivers in interpreting the baby's messages. Caregivers respond to the baby's cries, sounds, looks and gestures and imbue these behaviours with *communicative functions* such as protesting, requesting and rejecting. The mother of a crying 3-month-old baby may interpret her baby's cries as the baby 'wanting her nappy changed'. The fact that caregivers interpret young babies' communicative behaviours as intentional is considered by Trevarthen (1977) to make it possible for the baby to begin to communicate a wider range of messages in different ways.

Faces and voices

The focus of interaction between the very young baby and her mother is largely the emotional state of the other (Reddy 1999). There is a lot of evidence to suggest that babies are predisposed at birth to be interested in people and in particular in those features of people that are central to communication – faces and voices. There is additional evidence that very young babies respond appropriately to human communication in the form of imitation of facial expressions and some sounds (Meltzoff and Moore 1983, Kugiumutzakis 1993). Social motivation is evident in newborns, who engage in face-to-face interaction and who are more responsive to the human voice than to other sounds, and to the human face than other visual stimuli (Fantz 1963, Ashmead and Lipsitt 1977). This increases in complexity over the next few weeks. Back and forth games of 'vocal tennis' between babies and carers emerge by 3 months, and by 6 months of age the baby is able to look in the same direction as an adult's gaze, which results in 'joint reference' to the same objects and events in the environment (Butterworth 1991). Active participation in the establishment of joint reference occurs at 8 to 9 months of age when babies start to show, give and then point to objects as a form of social exchange. As outlined above, babies come to realize that through their own actions they can get other people to do things (Bates 1976).

The role of early interactive games

Early interactive games involving manipulation of controlled surprise such as peekaboo and tickling games come into their own half way through the first year. In the early stages of playing peekaboo, the baby's behaviour is predominantly passive. She hears the words and sees her mother's face disappearing and reappearing from behind her hands, for example. As the game is repeated many times the baby gradually learns to anticipate what happens in the game and her mother's expectations about her baby's responses in the game change. The baby is expected to take more of an active part in the game. The pattern of the game develops in line with the increasing demands made of the baby in terms of her responses. Where the baby first looks expressionlessly at her mother's face reappearing from behind her hands, she then chortles excitedly, then says 'boo!' without waiting for her mother to say it first, and finally initiates various adaptations of the game in a variety of settings. The baby becomes more systematic in how she communicates during these games, enabling her to take an ever more active part. She is motivated to play the games through her enjoyment of the rewarding element of controlled surprise played out with her mother.

The shift that takes place in the mother–child unit's communicative style from gentle vocalizations and close face-to-face interaction in the early months to the more boisterous, rhythmic baby songs around 6 months reflects in part the adult's need to maintain the baby's interest and attention (Reddy 1999). At this stage the baby becomes increasingly interested in her environment and is likely to look away from caregivers as other stimuli distract her.

Interest in objects

Between the 8th and 11th months the baby starts showing interest in exchanging objects with others and involving them in interaction with caregivers (Wellman 1993). Examples of these might be toys, food and interesting things to look at such as lights, the baby's reflection in the mirror and dogs on the street. The focus of interaction has shifted from the emotional states of the two partners during the earliest months, to the activity involved in the interactions around 6 months and now towards involving a third party (Reddy 1999). The move towards behaviours characteristic of this stage is gradual (Harding 1983, Wetherby and Prizant 1989). These behaviours include:

- the baby making eye contact with the partner in interaction while gesturing or vocalizing, often shifting gaze between an object and the partner (Bates 1979)
- more consistency in the sounds and intonation patterns of the baby's vocalizations
- pointing at objects which develops out of reaching towards them
- after vocalizing or making a gesture, the baby may then wait for a response from the partner.

Caregivers frequently infer from these behaviours that the baby is making requests for objects and directing the caregiver's attention to objects. As well as giving, requesting and showing, babies at this stage engage in showing off, following another's gaze, teasing and gazing at caregivers' facial expressions to guide further actions (social referencing) (Reddy 1999). Each of these behaviours indicates that the baby is developing an understanding of other people's attentional and emotional reactions. See page 34 for further discussion on these developments.

Example 1.2 Drawing another's attention towards a shared focus

Around the age of 9 months, Rowan started pointing at things and saying 'Da' as she did so. Sometimes she would alternate eye gaze between what had caught her attention and her mother. This usually resulted in her mother responding in some way, as in the conversation below. Here, Rowan succeeds in initiating and maintaining interaction through directing her mother's attention towards a light that had caught her interest.

ROWAN: *(pointing at light)* Da.
            (looks at her mother) Da.
MOTHER: What is it? The light? *(looks towards the light)*
ROWAN: *(pointing at light)* Da.
MOTHER: Da!

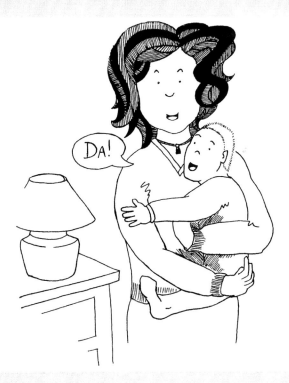

Figure 1.2 Nine-month-old Rowan draws her mother's attention towards something of interest

Enjoyable conversations as a context for the baby's developing communication skills

Early turn-taking

The development of turn-taking is fundamental to social interaction and to the development of conversations. A conversation, at its most basic, is a series of turns taken by more than one participant in interaction (Snow 1986). The turns taken may consist of looks, smiles, frowns, gestures, vocalizations, single words or complete sentences. In her first year, the baby has many opportunities to practice turn-taking with an adult caregiver. The beginning of conversational turn-taking is observed in the 'gaze coupling' of infants and caregivers (Jaffe *et al.* 1973). Mothers and very young infants have been observed by Snow (1977) to engage in vocal or verbal turn alternations. Snow (1977), Trevarthen (1980) and Lock (1993) place special significance on the caregiver's responses in early infant conversations, in that they behave as if the child has uttered actual words and thus share in the construction of meaning. In Halliday's scenario below, the mother is holding the baby in her lap and throwing and catching a stuffed rabbit while the child watches attentively.

> Mother: There he goes!
> Child: Ooh Ooh Ooh.
> Mother: Oh, you want me to throw him up again, do you? All right, there he
>   goes!
> Child: (Loudly) Mmng.
> Mother: No, that's enough. Let's find something else to do.
>
> (Halliday 1994: 73)

The mother does most of the talking but she accepts the child's response as legitimate in the turn-taking ritual. As the child grows and makes more intelligible utterances, the mother transfers more of the responsibility for continuing the dialogue to the child. The turn-taking ritual provides for optimal learning as the caregiver continues to model the language and support the deduction of meaning.

Responding to intonation and pauses

The way caregivers of very young babies interact with them is considered by Locke (1993) to help the development of communication. Extremes of vocal pitch serve to attract and maintain a baby's attention (Stern *et al.* 1982). Caregivers often use squeaky, high-pitched voices with a questioning intonation pattern when addressing babies. After saying something such as 'Hiya!! Baby girl!! Hiyaaa!' in this way, the adult will usually pause. The purpose of the pause is thought to allow the baby to take her turn (Stern *et al.* 1982). The baby may then smile, or look at the adult, or burp. The caregiver may then respond with, 'Oh, smiler!' or 'Does that feel better?', thus laying the foundations of conversational turn-taking which are increasingly strengthened over the forthcoming months. This type of response is seen by some writers as filling in the gaps in the baby's communicative competence

(Trevarthen 1980) while others (Reddy 1999) may argue for the child to be understood as a more equal, competent participant in early infant conversations. Either way, it is inescapable that the neonate, the young infant and the older baby engage in communication, albeit within observable limitations at each stage, in mutual partnership with another, driven by a strong sense of social motivation and a powerful interest in those aspects of communication that are particular to our species.

How babies communicate: looking, moving and gesturing

Babies and adults use looking, body movements and gestures to communicate with each other long before the baby develops verbal language. How babies move their bodies, their gaze, smiles, cries and other sounds are all important in developing interaction and evoking responses in their caregivers. Development of the social smile that occurs around 4 to 6 weeks is a cornerstone in social interaction and elicits many positive comments from caregivers.

Example 1.3 Interaction between a mother and infant

At 2 months, Rowan's nonverbal behaviours and focus of attention provide the content of interaction between herself and her mother.

ROWAN: *(smiles)*
MUM: Ooh, smiler. Are you a smiler, then? Smiley girl. There.
ROWAN: *(gaze wanders to the light in the corner)*
MUM: Are you looking at the light? Nice light . . . mmm.
ROWAN: *(burps)*
MUM: Ooh, burpy girl. Does that feel better now?

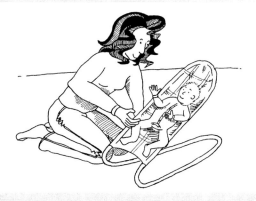

Figure 1.3 Two-month-old Rowan and her mother enjoy smiling at each other

---

The development of joint attention

Looking

Awareness of another person's direction of gaze and the development of eye contact with another are fundamental to joint interactions and are considered to underlie later conversational skills and the ability to see things from another person's perspective. At birth babies orient to other people by maintaining face-to-face gaze. At 2 months, babies meet the eye gaze of the person looking at them and by 3 months they look for and make contact with the other person's eyes (Bzoch and League 1991). At 4 months the baby initiates further interaction through eye contact and starts to develop joint attention with her mother by following her gaze (Ruddy and Bornstein 1988, Prizant and Wetherby 1990). You can see how Rowan's mother was keen to establish a joint focus of attention (the light) with her baby, thus helping her to learn about sharing focus on a topic (which can be elaborated on later). By 6 months the baby will look at the same object her mother is looking at and will begin to look at nearby objects her mother is pointing at (Butterworth and Jarrett 1991). At 9 months she will look at more distant objects her mother is pointing at (Bzoch and League 1991).

Moving and gesturing

Around this age many other behaviours that have started to emerge come together against the backdrop of the baby's increased understanding of other people's attentions and emotions. These behaviours include responding to gestures with gestures, for example waving bye-bye, kissing and clapping, and being guided by other people's gestures and facial expression. Early random arm movements made by the 3-month-old baby develop into grasping and reaching in the 6-month-old (Sheridan 1997). Pointing develops along with other gestures around 9 months and may occur together with vocalization to convey a request for an interesting object. These gestures include waving, reaching, raising arms, tugging and shaking the head.

Figures 1.4 to 1.9 illustrate the changing content and focus of interaction between the baby and caregiver at different points in the baby's development.

Using communication as a means to an end

Babies use behaviours such as looking, gesture, sounds or early *word approximations* in varying combinations to establish a shared focus of attention with somebody else and perform a range of communicative functions, in particular showing objects and pointing to objects and events they observe. Whatever her message, the important point is that well into the last quarter of her first year, the baby has learned that communication is an effective, pleasurable way to influence those around her and a way to exert some control over her environment.

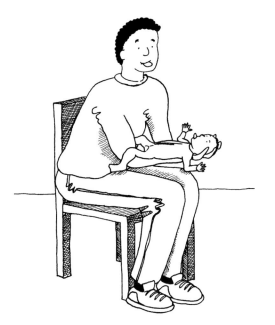

Figure 1.4 Six-week-old baby and father imitating each other's facial expressions. In the first few weeks of the baby's life, the content of interaction between the baby and caregiver focuses largely on the emotional state of the other. There is a high level of face-to-face interactions where actions such as vocalizations, smiles and other facial expressions in one partner often elicit similar actions in the other.

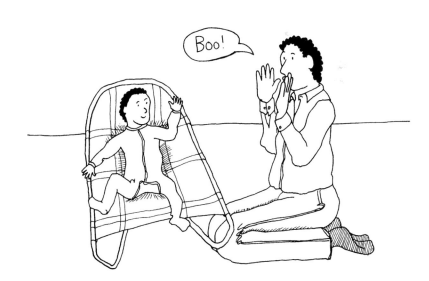

Figure 1.5 Six-month-old baby playing peekaboo with his father. Around 6 months, caregivers start to engage babies in interactive games such as peekaboo and 'This little piggy', involving manipulation of controlled surprise by the caregiver and anticipation in the baby. While a large part of the interaction continues to be face-to-face, the content of interaction also includes routines based around these repeated rhymes and games.

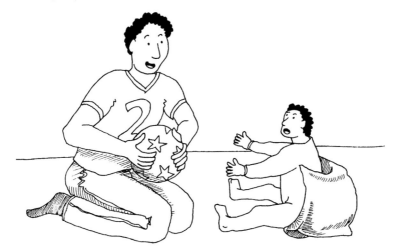

Figure 1.6 Father gives a ball to his 9-month-old baby. From about 8 months the baby starts showing interest in involving objects, for example toys in interaction between himself and his caregiver. He might, for example, hold a piece of biscuit or a ball to 'show' to his caregiver, but make no comment about it as such. Caregivers also show things to the baby, and exchange of objects (for example food and toys) becomes a focus of interaction.

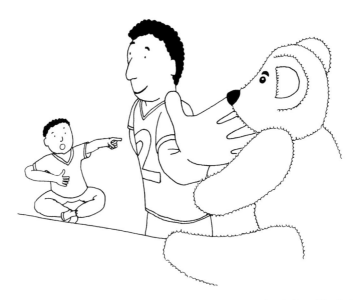

Figure 1.7 Eleven-month-old baby makes known his wish to his father. The baby might vocalize and/or gesture at a toy. He might then turn to look at his caregiver's face, alternating eye gaze between the toy and the caregiver's face. This results in the caregiver's attention being drawn to the toy, which is then given to the baby.

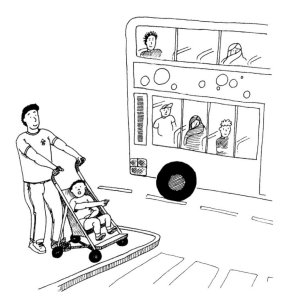

Figure 1.8 The baby draws his caregiver's attention to things. The baby vocalizes and/or gestures at an object. He then might turn to look at his caregiver's face, alternating eye gaze between the toy and his caregiver. The result is that the caregiver's attention is drawn to the object. This 11-month-old baby succeeds in drawing his father's attention towards the bus.

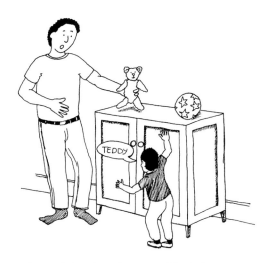

Figure 1.9 A 1-year-old uses words to ask for things he wants. The baby utters a word ('teddy') or word approximation ('de . . . de . . .') in reference to his focus of attention. He then might turn to look at his caregiver's face, alternating gaze between the teddy and his caregiver. The caregiver's attention is drawn to the baby's focus of attention (teddy), which may result in the caregiver giving the teddy to the baby.

Example 1.4 Using communication to influence others

At 5 months, Rowan cried and looked away from the loaded spoon at dinner time. She was not yet aware that these behaviours were responsible for causing any change – she might have been responding to her feeling of fullness, or lack of interest in the food, or desire to breastfeed. . . . Her mother, however, interpreted these behaviours as signs that her child did not want any more food. Five months later, if indeed this is what Rowan wants to communicate, she is well equipped to do so. She can shake her head, push the spoon away and make sounds of protest because she knows that by behaving in this way she can bring about some change. She can also say 'nononono'. As a result of these behaviours, Rowan may well be lifted out of her highchair, bringing an early conclusion to her meal.

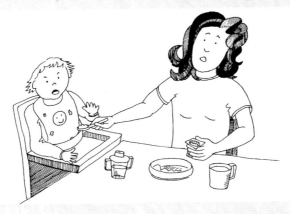

Figure 1.10 Ten-month-old Rowan is able to protest effectively when she does not want something

Making sounds in the first year

Crying

Crying is babies' earliest means of communicating their needs to their parents. Crying may be in response to the baby's internal physical state (for example hunger, pain, discomfort) or because they are upset, angry, lonely or frustrated. As babies' movement and language skills develop, their reliance on crying to signal their needs to parents decreases. Parents who find it particularly hard to cope with a crying baby, especially new or isolated parents, may benefit from being put in touch with other parents through organizations such as the National Childbirth Trust (see 'Useful Addresses', page 222). The opportunity to meet other parents in similar situations can be informative and supportive.

Special cries?

Some parents come to recognize the 'special' cries their babies make in response to different states, such as hunger – for others it can be more difficult to discriminate between cries. It can be very hard, especially for a new mother, to detect why a baby is crying. Perhaps the baby signals that she is hungry again just an hour after feeding, or maybe she is a baby who continues to cry, in spite of all her caregivers' sensitive and responsive attempts to comfort and tend to her. It is important to remember that like all people, babies are individuals and differ from each other in their behaviour and needs as we all do. For detailed information concerning the developmental and clinical significance of infant crying in the first few months and years of life, see Barr *et al.* (2000) and Lester and Zachariah Boukydis (1985). A summary of the different types of cry and of common causes for crying in babies appears in the following paragraphs.

Hunger, discomfort, pain, tiredness, irritation and boredom

Hunger cries are typically rhythmical: cry, breathe, cry, and may be preceded by little grunts and whimpers (Stark *et al.* 1975). Cries in response to pain are characteristically high pitched, often with sudden shifts in pitch (Stark *et al.* 1975). The onset of the cry is sudden and babies hold their breath for what can seem like an age between each cry. Discomfort cries do not have the loudness and sharp quality of pain cries and the duration of each expulsion of air within the cry is generally shorter than in other cries.

Most babies do not like being cold and some object to being dressed and undressed which can involve a lot of pulling about. Other causes of crying include feeling lonely, being over-stimulated, over-tired and frustrated. Babies, especially very young ones, need to be in close physical proximity to their caregivers; being alone can make them feel insecure until they are picked up and held. Very bright lights or very loud sounds can upset babies as their sensory systems find it hard to cope with such intense input.

Over-tiredness is a common, but often over-looked, cause of crying. Most parents do come to recognize the signs, especially as babies get older and their cries take on a whining quality. Early on, however, it can be very hard for parents to interpret the cries of an over-tired baby, particularly of babies whose sleep requirements change significantly through the weeks, for example during growth spurts.

Babies like to have things to do: they like to watch mobiles dance in the air and become entranced by geometric patterns and pictures of faces (Olson and Sherman 1983). Later, they like to make things happen, such as producing noises with rattles. Babies whose dummies have temporarily been taken away from them may cry with irritation. They may cry with frustration if their developing but limited motor skills prevent them from achieving goals such as reaching out to touch interesting objects. Clumsy movements, slowness or inability to move away from the position a baby is in might thwart her ambitions and bring forth tears of frustration.

Fear

Babies of 7 months and older may also cry from fear of strangers (Emde *et al.* 1976). Development of fear signals an important emotional and intellectual step and may manifest in sudden intense crying when a baby is held out to a stranger's arms or when an over-enthusiastic friend brings his face slightly too close for the baby's comfort. Where previously she accepted being passed to others to be held without protest, by 10 months and possibly before then she will have worked out what and who is familiar and belongs in her environment, and what and who does not (Sroufe *et al.* 1974). Anything or anyone who is not part of her familiar world is likely to be treated suspiciously; if familiar people leave her with someone unfamiliar, or if she finds herself in a very unfamiliar situation, she may become anxious and start to cry.

Crying beyond the first year

Babies and older children will continue to use crying as an important means of communicating with caregivers in many situations. As a baby's sensory, motor, cognitive and social skills develop so too do her communication skills. As adults listen, understand and respond to her cries in these early months they are laying the foundation for responsive communication to take place as the child gets older and uses more complex methods of communicating.

From vocalizing to babbling

The influence of changing anatomy on sound production

The range of sounds produced by humans is closely linked to anatomical structure, which develops over time (Bosma *et al.* 1965). At birth the space inside the mouth is small and almost totally filled with the baby's tongue (see Figure I.2, page 7). Also, the voice box is positioned fairly high up in the throat, which affects the timbre of the voice. The rapid growth of the baby's head and neck over the next few weeks and months leads to more varied types of sounds being produced.

Vegetative sounds

Most very young babies use their voices in the first eight weeks or so of life not only to cry but also to make a range of other sounds. In the first eight weeks babies sigh and grunt, especially when active in some way (Stark 1986). They fuss when not particularly comfortable, burp, blow raspberries, let out short squeals and might say a few vowel-type sounds such as 'ee', 'oo' and 'aa'. In the very early weeks, these sounds are usually a lead-in to crying. As babies get a bit older they come to use these sounds, termed by Stark as vegetative sounds, at other times, especially when happy.

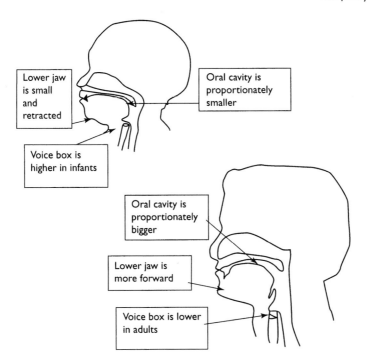

Figure 1.11 Anatomical differences between the adult's and baby's oral and pharyngeal structures

Table 1.1 Summary of vocal development from birth to 6 months

Summary of vocal development from birth to 6 months	
Birth	Cries and vegetative sounds
2 months	Coos and gurgles
4 months	Vocal play – squeals, yells, trills
6 months	Babbles

Cooing and gurgling

Around 8 weeks, babies start to *gurgle* and *coo*, especially in response to friendly faces and people talking to them (Stark 1986). Cooing and gurgling sounds are made when the muscles at the back of the mouth in the throat and soft palate make intermittent contact with the back of the tongue during longer vowel sounds. The sounds 'k' and 'g' can be identified in a baby's cooing – 'cooo . . .

gaaa' – giving the name to this stage of vocal development. Between 2 and 3 months, babies often respond to people talking or other sounds by vocalizing, sometimes with two or more different *syllables* together – 'aah eee khaa' (Bzoch and League 1991).

Laughter and vocal play

From 12 weeks onwards there is a marked decrease in crying, and sustained laughter emerges at about 16 weeks (Stark 1986). For the next two months or so, babies engage in '*vocal play*'. Loud yells, high pitched squeals and low pitched growls, lip smacking, blowing 'raspberries', a wider range of vowels and some consonant/ vowel sequences such as 'mmmuh', 'uhn' characterize this period. Sounds such as 'b', 'p', 't' and 'd' occur, along with prolonged vowel sounds. The wide range of sounds produced in vocal play are transitional between the comforting cooing sounds of earlier days and the sounds of true babbling which emerge around 6 months (Stark 1986). The baby makes the sounds of vocal play in a variety of communicative situations, for example in back and forth vocalization games with adults which she often initiates, and when looking at or reaching for something or someone she wants (Bzoch and League 1991). This last example might be interpreted by caregivers as the baby making a request for the thing she wants, or for the person to do something such as pick her up. Adults no longer have to rely on the baby's cry to tell whether she is angry but can do so by listening to her vocalizations, which also tell if she is pleased about something.

From babbling to early words

The functions of babbling

The strings of repeated consonant/vowel and vowel sequences constituting what most people think of as babbling – 'mamama', 'bababa', 'nununu', 'dadada' – start to emerge around 6 months (Locke 1993). Locke suggests that babbling represents functional integration of increased articulatory motor control and sensory feedback systems. Babbling may occur in response to social stimulation, as with earlier cooing, but many babies babble more when they are on their own in a self-stimulatory manner (Stark 1986). Ritual imitation babbling games that develop out of parents responding to their babies' babbling by babbling back, are considered to help babies further on their path towards speech. Auditory feedback of the baby's own sounds is thought to play an important role in promoting the development of babbling. The range of consonant sounds that babies use most in babbling at this stage is restricted and includes those that occur in their early words a few months later (Locke 1993). This is true for babies worldwide, of all languages. Locke cites several studies demonstrating a significant degree of continuity between the sounds produced in babbling and sounds of speech produced by older babies and children at the early stages of talking. He suggests that one of the functions of babbling is to provide the baby with a range of 'speech-like syllables and segments [sounds] that it elaborates prior to and during the development of an expressive lexicon [vocabulary]' (Locke 1993: 208). While speech does not develop directly from babble, the onset of babbling indicates a state of neurological development that is in readiness for speech to begin. Babies enjoy babbling; babbling is a form of play and is thus considered to be a sign of a healthy, happy baby (Locke 1993).

The transition towards purposeful use of sounds

Babies continue to take turns with others in producing sounds and now listening attentively for the response. When they are about 7 months, babies vocalize about half the time when called by their name (Bzoch and League 1991). When looking at a person a baby may make a range of sounds, with changes in loudness and pitch of the voice together with smiling and body movements. Adults might interpret these behaviours as the baby showing interest and awareness in other people.

Around 8 months babies make sounds and some gestures related to speech action games like 'Pat-a-cake', 'Peekaboo' and 'Row your boat' which might be interpreted by adults as the baby requesting one or other of the games. These are examples of speech action games played by English-speaking families; variations along the same themes are found universally. Babies now begin to use their voices to attract attention from others, for example yelling loudly if in a different room to an adult (Bzoch and League 1991).

Jargon

Around 9 months, babies start to combine different consonants and vowels in their babble and the range of consonants used increases to include sounds like 'g', 's' and other 'hissing' sounds like 'ch' in 'loch' (Stark 1986). It may sound like 'bahboo . . . amayooo . . . wiyoh . . .' and is known as '*jargon*'. The stretches of jargon can be quite long, like sentences, and from a short distance away it might sound as if the baby is actually speaking in sentences. In addition to imitating other people's voices and the intonation pattern of sentences heard around her, the baby uses a variety of intonation patterns in her jargon which can sound as if she is speaking a foreign language. At this age babies may use jargon when they look at pictures in books, when playing with the telephone and in general play. It might be possible for adults to catch a real word among the jargon and short exclamations such as 'Ooh!'

Sound imitation games

Ritualized sound imitation games with adults are common at this stage. For example, the adult says a sound such as 'Mmmhmm', which the baby then imitates, which is then imitated by the adult in turn, and so on. Turn-taking in these games can go on for a very long time. The baby will also enjoy taking turns in speech-action games and play with toys with looks, actions, sounds and gestures (Bzoch and League 1991).

Protowords

Some writers (Bates *et al.* 1975) place significant focus on the observation that the baby at this stage is communicating with a goal in mind – her communication is clearly 'intentional' and she becomes very sociable. She makes functional use of certain sounds as if they were words, as Phoebe's use of 'Ugh!' combined with looking and pointing at an object was used to mean 'Give me that!' A baby's consistent use of a sound in this way is idiosyncratic and does not necessarily bear any relation to the surrounding language. These functional, consistent sound patterns have variably been termed *'protowords'* and *'vocables'* by researchers (Dore *et al.* 1976, Ferguson 1978). She may 'ask' questions such as 'Who's that?' by pointing at someone while saying a sound with a questioning intonation.

Words emerge

By around 12 months the baby may well be producing some words that are recognizable forms of words from the adult language (Bloom and Lahey 1978, Locke 1993). Characteristically, the way the baby pronounces the same word will be slightly different on different occasions (Stackhouse and Wells 1997). For example, between the ages of 11 and 15 months, Rowan's pronunciations of the word 'pear' included: 'bear', 'bah', 'buh', 'boh', 'pear' and 'pah' amongst many others. This characteristic of early word pronunciations tells us that children's motor control for speech has a way to go before stable pronunciations can be expected (Stackhouse and Wells 1997). The rate of vocabulary development varies enormously between children and is discussed in the next chapter.

Overlap between stages of sound production and continuity of nonverbal communication

It is important to realize that there is considerable overlap between each of the stages outlined above. Children who are in the early stages of using real words do not suddenly stop babbling or using jargon. Emergence of conventional gestures such as pointing occurs around 9 months when babies are babbling and jargoning; pointing continues into adulthood, long after the establishment of real words, to support what a speaker says, or indeed to supplement spoken language.

Summary of Chapter 1

Hearing, attention and listening

1 Babies' hearing is well developed (though not completely) at birth. There is evidence to suggest babies are predisposed to listen to the human voice, in particular that of their mother.
2 Babies become more selective over the first year in what they attend to and by the end of the first year listen attentively to speech.

Towards early verbal understanding

3 Babies develop concepts about objects, events and people in their world through experience and play. Children need to have concepts of objects before they can link verbal labels to them.
4 Aspects of the situation in which language is spoken give crucial information supporting the baby's developing verbal understanding.

Communication and expressive skills in the first year: why do babies communicate?

5 From their earliest moments, babies display social motivation. This provides a context for communication skills to develop.
6 Babies show particular interest in species-specific aspects of communication carried by faces and voices.
7 There is a gradual shift in the focus of interaction between the baby and her mother over the first year from each other's emotional states, to the activity of interaction games, to objects such as interesting toys or food.
8 Towards the end of the first year, the baby comes to learn that she can use her communication skills in pleasurable and purposeful ways to bring about changes in her environment.

How babies communicate: looking, moving and gesturing

9 Babies gradually learn about other people having feelings and a focus of attention, and gradually increase their ability to share a focus of attention with others.
10 Various combinations of looking, moving, gesturing and vocalizing assist babies towards the end of the first year in directing another person's attention towards what they are interested in.

Making sounds in the first year

11 Crying is the baby's earliest way of signalling to her mother that something is wrong, and is therefore an important means of communication.
12 Sound production is partly influenced by the baby's developing anatomy.
13 *Vegetative sounds* are made in the first eight weeks and are followed by cooing and gurgling, then vocal play and laughter around 12 weeks.
14 After around six months, babies combine sounds in babble. Jargon follows on, with emergence of protowords and real word towards the end of the first year.

Key skills 1.1 Communication skills usually achieved by 3-month-old babies

- Cries
- Smiles at people, toys
- Looks at people, toys
- Makes eye contact
- Briefly grasps object placed in her hand
- Makes vowel-type sounds
- Coos and gurgles
- Startle response to loud, sudden noise
- Responds to speech by looking at speaker's face

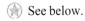 See below.

Key skills 1.2 Communication skills usually achieved by 6-month-old babies

- Appears to understand tones of warning, anger and friendliness in voices
- Seems to recognize names of family members
- Recognizes own name
- Takes part in back-and-forth vocalization games with adults
- Some consonants (for example b, p, t, d and a range of vowels) are included in early babble
- Looks at what an adult is looking at
- Participates in turn-taking games like pat-a-cake
- Explores objects by looking and touching
- Very interested in looking at what people are doing

Before using these tables, see page xxi.

Key skills 1.3 Communication skills usually achieved by 9-month-old babies

- Stops activity when her name is called
- Looks towards speaker who calls her name
- Stops activity in response to 'no'
- Tuneful babble with a range of consonants
- Gestures (usually points) and vocalizes to request things
- Looks at objects pointed at by others
- Gives objects to another person on request
- Performs routine activities on request (for example waves 'bye-bye')
- Understands names of a few very common objects in her environment

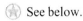 See below.

Key skills 1.4 Communication skills usually achieved by 12-month-old babies

- Understands several object names
- Responds appropriately to some verbal requests
- Makes appropriate verbal responses to some requests (for example, 'Say bye-bye')
- 'Talks' to people and toys in long tuneful stretches
- Uses one to three words or word approximations with a degree of consistency
- Vocalizes in response to being spoken to
- Uses combination of looking, gesture and vocalization or word/word approximation to make requests, comment or protest
- Demonstrates appropriate but fleeting use of toys and objects (for example, touches comb to hair with tines facing up; puts blanket on doll in crib but only covers doll's face)

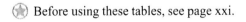 Before using these tables, see page xxi.

Warning signs 1.1 Possible warning signs for 3-month-old babies

- **Does not smile**
- **Is not vocalizing**
- **Does not cry to signal hunger or pain**
- **Never turns her head towards sounds**
- **Parents express concerns, are worried or anxious**

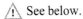 See below.

Warning signs 1.2 Possible warning signs for 6-month-old babies

- **Does not look towards speakers**
- **Does not visually track moving objects**
- **Does not babble using consonant and vowel sounds (for example 'Ma', 'ba', 'goo')**
- **Is quiet, apart from crying**
- **Parents express concerns, are worried or anxious**

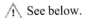 See below.

Warning signs 1.3 Possible warning signs for 9-month-old babies

- **Is not interested in socially interactive games (for example peek-aboo)**
- **Does not recognize her own name**
- **Does not make many sounds**
- **Does not produce strings of babble (for example 'Mamamama', 'babababab', 'gagagagaga')**
- **Is not interested in toys that make noises**
- **Parents express concerns, are worried or anxious**

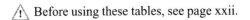 Before using these tables, see page xxii.

Warning signs 1.4 Possible warning signs for 12-month-old babies

- **Does not identify familiar objects when they are named**
- **Does not turn her head towards the speaker when her name is called**
- **Does not produce lots of tuneful babble**
- **Does not look in the direction of a pointing finger**
- **Parents express concerns, are worried or anxious**

⚠ Before using this table, see page xxii.

The second year

- ○ Key stages of language development and links with developments in play, cognition, attention and listening.
- ○ Development of communication skills in the second year and reasons for communicating.
- ○ Summary of key points; tables of communication skills usually achieved in the second year; tables of possible warning signs to help identify children with communication difficulties.

Attention and learning language

During the second year of life, children can attend to an activity that they have chosen, such as a puzzle, for variable periods of time (Reynell 1980). They may be able to attend to some activities for extended durations on some occasions, displaying a very short attention span on others. At the start of the second year, the ability to attend to a task is highly unstable, resulting in the child displaying rigid and inflexible attention in the need to ignore extraneous stimuli. Children at this stage find it hard to respond to either visual or verbal intervention, or to attempts by others to modify their task. They might be labelled 'stubborn' or even suspected to be deaf due to the *single-channelled* nature of their attention (Reynell 1980). The ability to attend and respond to language spoken to them while engaged in an activity depends enormously on whether the words spoken relate intrinsically to the activity or not. This is related to the single-channelled nature of attention at this stage; integration of visual, verbal and tactile sources of information occurs at a later stage.

It is well documented that children in their second year vary enormously in both the number and type of words they use (Nelson 1981, cited by Tomasello and Todd 1983: 198). Studies by Tomasello and colleagues (Tomasello and Todd 1983, Tomasello and Farrar 1986) have contributed to explaining this fact. These have focused on the interplay between maternal interactional style, attentional factors in children and their learning of object names. Tomasello and Todd (1983) found that differences in the ability of pairs of mothers and their children (aged 15 to 21 months) in establishing and maintaining a joint focus of attention were related to the child's subsequent language growth. Mannle and Kruger (1986), cited by Tomasello and Farrar (1986), found that the amount of time mothers and children spent in episodes involving a joint focus of attention at 15 months was positively correlated with vocabulary size at 21 months. Early nonverbal joint interactions around a shared focus of attention have thus been found to provide support for children's early verbal interactions (Tomasello and Farrar 1986). This effect was found to continue well into the second half of the second year.

Tomasello and Todd (1983) report that when mothers name objects that are already within a child's focus of attention, the child is more likely to be able to link the names of objects with their *referents*, resulting in greater language development at 21 months. Thus, children of mothers who use a child-centred interactional style when introducing words to their children, learn more words. The factor relating to maternal interactional style was found to be a strong determinant of subsequent word learning by children, rather than other factors relating to the type of words introduced. Mothers who say words to their children as they are directing their attention to something new are less likely to establish the shared attentional focus with their child necessary for learning a word. When mothers attempt to redirect a child's attention when naming an object, the child needs to shift her attention so as to coordinate with the adult's if she is to succeed in matching the object name with the object. As outlined in the previous paragraph, it is extremely difficult for children of this age to shift attention in this manner. Adult directiveness in the form of verbal or nonverbal attempts to direct a child's attention or behaviour was found to be negatively correlated with the proportion of names for objects in a child's vocabulary at 21 months (Tomasello and Todd 1983).

Play and symbolic understanding

Children's play in the second year reflects their developing understanding about the world, their *symbolic understanding* and *conceptual categorization*. While certain cognitive skills may not necessarily be prerequisites for language development (Paul 1995), certain play behaviours are frequently observed to accompany particular communicative developments. *Representational play* is play with objects according to their functions and what they represent. Paul (1995) cites a study by Bates, Bretherton, Snyder, Shore and Volterra (1980) which revealed an association during the *single-word* period between the use of words as labels and early representational play using objects outside of the normal context for their conventional purposes, such as using a comb or spoon appropriately in play. At 1 year old, children begin to handle objects differentially. Spoons go into mouths, toy cars are pushed along and dolls are held. This differential treatment reflects children's developing ability to categorize objects. Carers have been observed to label objects according to how children appear to categorize them – this has the partial effect of showing how words relate to objects.

Example 2.1 Adult labels reflect the child's categorization of the world

At 14 months, Ruby showed her mother a toy warthog and snorted as she was used to doing when seeing real pigs, playing with toy pigs and seeing pictures of pigs. Her mother said, 'Yes, that's a pig. Oink oink.' By saying this, Ruby's mother 'colludes' in Ruby's rudimentary categorization development, labelling the toy according to Ruby's current category framework.

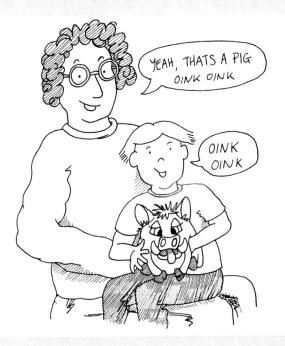

Figure 2.1 Fourteen-month-old Ruby shows her mother a toy warthog

Half-way through the second year, children sort toys and objects into gross categories such as people, animals and food. They sort by colour around the same age. Representational play develops so that by 14 months the child pretends at simple activities such as brushing hair and talking on the telephone. This is followed shortly by simple sequenced *pretend play* that might involve making a cup of tea, scraping out a bowl with a spoon and then feeding a doll with the spoon. There are of course many other developments in play, but included here are those aspects of play that are most closely linked to language development. A bit later, when children start to *combine words*, they also start to produce sequences of actions in play, such as pretending to feed and bathe a doll. Symbolic development occurs gradually through the course of the second year. A symbol is something that 'stands for' something else, such as a toy cup or a picture of a cup, which can represent the

Table 2.1 Stages of symbolic understanding in the second year

Age range	Stage of symbolic development	Play behaviour
12 to 14 months	*Object recognition:* Concepts of objects become decontextualized beyond particular situations to all objects which are perceptually similar. So, the concept a child has of her own sponge at bath time is generalized to any real-sized sponge in any context. This stage occurs immediately prior to early symbolic understanding.	Brief but appropriate use of common objects such as combs, cups, brushes and spoons outside of the normal context: picks up a comb, touches it to hair, sets it aside, picks up the phone, puts it to ear, drops it.
15 to 18 months	*Large doll play:* Toys used in large doll play are closely related to daily living and represent objects for which children have developed object concepts. This level of representational play uses easy symbols which closely resemble the real objects.	Links two thematically related toys through actions. Early play sequences enacted: brushes doll's hair, feeds doll, places cup on plate, spoon in cup. Gradual increase in number and complexity of play sequences.
18 to 21 months	*Small doll play:* This level of representational play uses more difficult symbols. The toys used in small doll play are less closely linked perceptually to the objects they represent.	Links two or more thematically related toys through actions. Later play involves playing out sequences: feeding doll, bathing doll, putting doll to bed.
18 to 24 months	*Two-dimensional symbols:* Recognition of pictures. Pictures comprise the most difficult level of symbolic understanding in children of this age, bearing little perceptual similarity to the objects they represent. Simple colour photographs are the easiest form of picture to understand, bearing a closer resemblance to their referents than black and white photographs or drawings.	Matches real objects to pictures at first, later matches toys to pictures.

Sources: Paul (1995) and Cooper et al. (1978).

concept of a cup. Symbolic understanding gradually increases so that children are able to link increasingly arbitrary representations of objects and events to relevant concepts (Cooper *et al*. 1978). Stages of symbolic understanding and associated play behaviours that occur during the second year are outlined in Table 2.1, which draws on the work of Paul (1995) and Cooper *et al*. (1978).

Understanding meaning

In early stages of development children may only understand a particular word or phrase when spoken in a particular context and when accompanied by a gesture. As she enters her second year, the young child's understanding of speech addressed to her continues to develop, but remains largely context-bound (Myers Pease *et al*. 1989). She cannot yet be said to have acquired true verbal understanding, that is, the ability to identify an object or event purely by its verbal label without contextual support. Children at this stage appear to understand more words than they actually do by relying on their understanding of the situation and using *nonlinguistic strategies* to comprehend the language they hear. In a naturalistic setting, such as home, a child will need little or no verbal understanding to respond appropriately to an instruction such as, 'Put it in the bin', as illustrated in Example 2.2.

Language content

The content of language, or, what people talk about and what they understand of what other people say, is to do with objects and events in the world and the ideas, feelings and attitudes that they have about what they know (Bloom and Lahey 1978). What children talk about and what they understand of what others say draws from knowledge that is gradually stored in memory. Children's knowledge is affected by their changing abilities to think and feel about objects and events in their environments (Bloom and Lahey 1978). The capacity for verbal comprehension and verbal expression in young children is determined, then, by the knowledge available to them and the situational context they find themselves in. It is the interplay between knowledge and context that provides the content of language. Children need to learn the words that stand for elements of content in order for language to be meaningful. Learning the meanings of words enables children to express to other people the content of their minds.

Words as symbols

But what is a word? We can take the example of a child who learns the meaning of the word 'teddy'. The child's actual teddy bear is the referent (or, 'thing referred to') for the word teddy. There is nothing special about the sound or shape of the word that makes it a more appropriate name for such a toy – different languages have different words of different lengths and syllable shapes involving a range of sounds for the same toy. The relationship between the word and its referent is arbitrary and

Example 2.2 Use of nonlinguistic strategies

Early in her second year, Rowan was 'helping' her father to sweep the kitchen floor. She picked up a piece of toast and showed it to her father who pointed at the bin and said, 'Ooh, dirty. Put it in the bin.' Rowan promptly dropped the toast in the bin. She was able to carry out the instruction as she had learned that things picked up off the floor often get placed in the bin, her father pointed at the bin as he spoke, and she was holding the piece of toast about which she had initiated an interaction with her father. The sum of Rowan's nonlinguistic knowledge about the situation (putting things picked up off the floor in the bin) and her strategy of 'doing what you usually do' (Paul 1995), usually used by children this age under these circumstances, together with making use of her father's gestural cue and relating this knowledge to the piece of toast in her hand, meant that she was able to respond appropriately to the instruction.

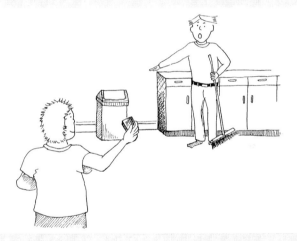

Figure 2.2 Early in her second year, Rowan follows her father's instruction

symbolic. Speakers of the same language implicitly agree to give particular names to different objects, events and actions. So in English a small, furry, cuddly toy with legs, arms and head somewhat resembling a bear is a 'teddy'. Not all words are symbolic, however. Onomatopoeic words such as 'splash' exist in English. Many of children's early words do not have a completely arbitrary relationship with their referents: cars are often called 'brrmbrrm', cows are 'moomoo' and dogs are 'woofwoof'. This may be because words that are obviously related to their referents are easier for young children to learn (Myers Pease *et al.* 1989).

The question now is, how do children in their second year come to understand and use words as symbols, to release them from the context in which they were first heard and so be able to use them creatively in a range of situations? The area of language development that is to do with developing an understanding of word meaning is called semantic development.

The role of context

Several factors are thought to influence early development of word meaning. As discussed, context is important. The more experiences a child has, the more opportunity she has for making observations about her world. As she has these experiences, carers talk about them with her. When she is ready, she can map the language she hears onto her understanding of the situation she has already developed through her repeated observations of repeated experiences. A young child who understands the meaning of 'bath time' may be responding to a range of situational cues in the early stages of her verbal comprehension. It may be the time of day when she expects to have her bath, she may see the water as it runs from the tap into the tub or her mother may be holding objects she associates with having a bath (sponge, towel, plastic duck). It can take a good deal of time before very young children are able to truly relate a verbal concept ('bath time') to a meaningful event (experience of warm soapy water in a tub accompanied by washing, sponges, soap and plastic ducks) and in any context (Bloom and Lahey 1978). Repeated experience accompanied by relevant talk from carers helps young children to make the link between the meanings of words and their referents.

Objects, concepts and words

In order for children to acquire the same meanings of words (and thus concepts of words) as adults, they need first to develop concepts of objects, events and relations between these which match adult concepts. The process of conceptual development that takes place over the second year can be compared in some ways to a process of ever greater differentiation and specification of the child's knowledge of herself and the world around her. Refer back to pages 25–26 for an introductory discussion on the development of object and relational concepts.

Information on how children at this age learn about objects, people and the relationships between them can be found in the errors they sometimes make when using words. These errors also provide information on how children learn about words. Children go through different stages of testing out their ideas about concepts and the meanings of words (*hypothesis testing*) until theirs correspond to and are consistent with those of mature speakers of the same language (Bloom and Lahey 1978).

Development of word knowledge

It is well reported that children in their second year use words in situations and to refer to the world around them in ways that do not always correspond with adults' use of the same words.

Just because a young child says a word is not reason enough to assume that she knows the word. Knowing the word 'teddy' involves:

- knowing that the word refers to a soft, furry toy with a face resembling that of a bear
- knowing that the word can be used to refer not only to the child's own teddy, but to all other teddies in the world, in a range of different locations and contexts
- knowing the meaning of the word when in combination with other words, for example knowing the difference between big teddy, small teddy, my teddy, Phoebe's teddy etc.
- knowing that teddy belongs to the category of words called toys due to shared features pertaining, in this case, to function, i.e. objects children use to play with.

The development in knowledge about words outlined above is implicit in the child, that is, she does not yet know that she knows what she does about words and hence the underlying object and relational concepts. It is important also to state that just because a child says a word appropriately in one context does not necessarily imply that she would be able to do so in different contexts. Development of word knowledge is gradual, starting around 12 months of age and continues well into the school years (Bloom and Lahey 1978).

Once a child has made a link between a word and some element of her experience she then proceeds to test out her understanding of the word's meaning by using it in a range of contexts. Feedback available from the environment in the form of adult responses to the words she says, for example, helps her to make the necessary adjustments to her concept of that word's meaning until it stabilizes. It is at this point that her concept of the word matches that of the adult. On her way to achieving a stable concept of a word, the child may employ a combination of strategies, some of which are outlined below.

Underextension and overextension of word meanings

During the early stages of single-word production, many children typically restrict their use of a word to a particular context – one that closely resembles the context in which they first made the link between the word and its referent. An example of this would be the child who uses the word 'ball' only to refer to her own ball. This is '*underextension*' of the word's meaning, using the adult meaning of the word as the standard. '*Overextension*' is where children try out, in a range of contexts, the meaning of a word they have learned, to find the best 'fit' (Bloom and Lahey 1978). An example of this is use of the word 'mummy' to refer to all women, including a child's own mother.

Using the same word for different meanings

During the first half of the second year, children have tentative concepts of objects in the world around them. This is reflected in the types of errors some children make in naming objects at this stage. The original context in which a child hears a word forms the basis for learning the word's meaning (Bloom and Lahey 1978). The child whose mother says, 'Let's put your shoes on' as she puts the child's shoes on may not differentiate between the other possible referents (socks, coat, hat, bag) which might be present in the same situation. That child might associate the word 'shoe' with any of these objects and subsequently erroneously name them as such. Resultant feedback from adults will then assist her in making an accurate match between the word 'shoe' and the appropriate object. For example, the child might point at her coat on a subsequent occasion and say 'Shoe'. Her mother may provide feedback by picking up a shoe and saying, 'Here's your shoe. Look, your shoe!' Another type of association the child could make is when she and her mother pass a shoe shop with lots of shoes in the window. She points at the shop window and says 'Shoe'. Her mother might applaud, giving positive feedback. The next time the child sees a different shop window, she may well point at it and say 'Shoe'. The objects are associated because the child experienced them together in a previous situation and did not differentiate between them for the meaning of the word, in this case, 'shoe'.

This type of association is representative of 'shifting connections among figurative, functional, and affective features of otherwise diverse objects and events' (Bloom and Lahey 1978: 122), and is more commonly reported in children who are still learning the underlying object and relational concepts of words.

Using the same word for related meanings

Towards the second half of the second year, children's word meanings are more consistently defined by the properties of the objects they represent. Children, especially early on, have many more concepts of objects than names of objects. At this stage, they make links between similar objects according to certain criteria. These are reported by Clark (1973), cited by Bloom and Lahey (1978), to relate to movement, texture, four-leggedness, shape and size. The words 'dog', 'bear', 'cat' and 'lion' all refer to objects that are animate, have four legs and fur. At an earlier stage when children are failing to differentiate between different objects (the animals listed above, for example), they may use a single word 'dog' to refer to them all. Later on, when children's object concepts are more stable and they are better able to differentiate between objects of different categories, yet are limited by a small vocabulary, they may use one word to refer to a set of objects either because they do not have the available vocabulary, or because they have made links between different object concepts (Bloom and Lahey 1978). It is not uncommon for parents to relate stories of their young child calling unfamiliar men 'daddy'. These children are overextending their conceptual category referred to as 'daddy' to include other men (or, as in Rowan's case in Example 2.3, just other men that look like her daddy).

Example 2.4 illustrates Rowan testing out her hypotheses of what the words 'woofwoof' and 'baabaa' mean. Her erroneous naming of the bear and poodle cannot be considered as random labelling, however. In each case, she had taken some preliminary information about what the words 'woofwoof' and 'baabaa' mean (information derived from previous experience of hearing and saying the words)

Example 2.3 Overextension of a conceptual category

At around 17 months, Rowan was shopping with her mother when suddenly she pointed at a man with a shaved head and said, 'Daddy!' Her father had just the previous week had his head similarly shaved. Rowan's behaviour did not suggest, however, that she thought this man was her father – she appeared instead to be commenting on the likeness in some way.

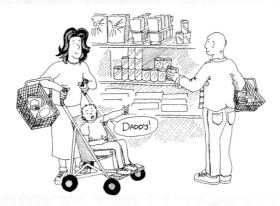

Figure 2.3 Seventeen-month-old Rowan calls a stranger 'Daddy'

and made a reasonable judgement that each word might fit a new situation. With the growth of vocabulary and consideration of environmental feedback to the words she uses, the child reorganizes her understanding of word meanings.

The errors that young children make in the names they give objects and events at this stage are informative for what they tell us about how children conceptually categorize knowledge they acquire about the world around them. During the second half of the second year, children's concepts of objects and events become progressively more stable (Bloom and Lahey 1978). In Example 2.4, Rowan demonstrates that she has made a link between her concepts for dogs and bears, and sheep and poodles (Example 2.4 describes Rowan's first sighting of a poodle). Bears and dogs have much in common – four legs, fluffy coats, wet noses – as do poodles and sheep – four legs, fluffy white coats. It is reasonable for a child developing her concepts of these animals to link them in this way. Presumably the picture of the bear that Rowan saw matched her current criteria for inclusion in her category of dogs, as the poodle matched her current criteria for sheep.

The young child's conceptual development and knowledge about categories helps her to link words that are associated in some way. This makes it easier to learn words that are grouped together such as 'sheep', 'dog', and 'bear'. When they are a bit older, children come to learn words that represent higher levels of categorization (for example 'animal', 'clothes', 'food') (Bancroft 1995).

Example 2.4 Naming errors reveal how early talkers categorize the world

At 14 months, Rowan had learned to associate the word 'woofwoof' with dogs. In a shop one day she saw a picture of a grizzly bear, which she pointed at and said 'woofwoof'. Shortly after this, she had learned to associate the word 'baabaa' with sheep. Out in the park a large fluffy white poodle scampered past her buggy – she pointed after it and said, 'baabaa'.

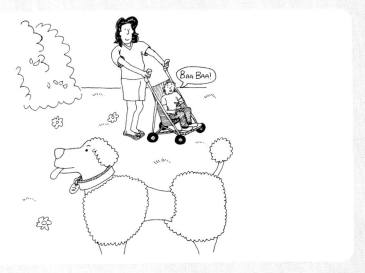

Figure 2.4 Fourteen-month-old Rowan calls a poodle 'baabaa'

Early verbal understanding

The stages of development of verbal language in children usually proceed according to a fairly consistent overall pattern (Cooper *et al.* 1978). The pattern of developmental stages is comparable for verbal comprehension and expressive language, but with the stages in verbal comprehension preceding the stages in expressive language.

12 to 18 months

Situational understanding of phrases

By 12 months a baby has developed good situational understanding of phrases, as outlined in Chapter 1 and this chapter. She shows an understanding of familiar phrases that occur as part of a routine, and responds appropriately. The baby who claps her hands as part of a game regularly played with her mother in response to the phrase 'Clap hands', for example, is taking part in a well-learned sequence of events and demonstrating an understanding which is bound to that particular context. Her response is due to the right person in the right situation saying the phrase using the right intonation and rhythm – the individual words have no meaning as yet.

Situational understanding of words within phrases

Soon into the second year the young child responds with appropriate actions to short phrases that signal a familiar routine (Cooper *et al.* 1978). For example, 'Shall we run the bath? Bath time!' will prompt her to stop what she is doing and possibly go towards the bathroom. She is beginning to understand the meanings of individual words (here, 'bath') spoken in phrases, but is still dependent on the phrases being uttered in a particular context. Questions such as 'Where's dolly?' may elicit a head turn in the right direction, but possibly only if she is in a situation where she expects to see her own doll. She might not yet have generalized the meaning of the word 'doll' to include other dolls.

True verbal understanding

Between approximately 12 and 15 months, children start to understand the labels of objects wherever the objects are, and understanding becomes far less dependent on a particular context, intonation pattern or speech rhythm (Cooper *et al.* 1978). Children are now acquiring true verbal understanding and are soon able to identify single objects in response to naming. For example a child should be able to select any doll (not just her own) from a choice of objects in front of her, when she hears the phrase 'Show me the doll', or 'Where's the doll?' A rapid spurt in the number of words that children understand occurs between 15 and 18 months (Bates *et al.* in press). Bates *et al.* cite a study by Fenson and colleagues (1994) where parents of 1,800 children in North America estimated their children to understand an average of 67 words at 10 months, 86 words at 12 months, 156 words at 14 months and 191 words at 16 months. Around 16 months, children are able to identify several body parts, such as 'eyes', 'nose', 'hands', 'toes', and understand some words other than names of objects or actions, such as 'in' and 'on'. By 18 months they can follow two-part instructions such as, 'Get the *bottle* and give it to *baby*' and can identify two familiar objects from a group of four or more familiar objects (Bzoch and League 1991).

18 to 24 months

Towards an understanding of complex sentences

During the second half of her second year, the young child becomes increasingly able to understand longer sentences. She can soon follow a series of two or three very simple but related commands such as 'Go to the *kitchen* and get your *beaker* from the *table*'. She combines her understanding of nonlinguistic information to supplement her knowledge of language, thus appearing at times to have more sophisticated verbal comprehension than might be the case. Children make use of *comprehension strategies* which allow them to combine information from gestures, facial expression and the way things usually happen with their understanding of the meanings of words (Paul 1995). At a minimum, a child needs to understand the meanings of the words 'kitchen' and 'beaker' from the above command in order to successfully carry out the instruction. Children at this age know that adults often ask them to do things; the child in question probably connects the kitchen as the place where her beaker is usually located; on entering the kitchen the child may immediately see the beaker on the table and thus not need to understand the meaning of that word in order to carry out the instruction.

The child's increasing understanding of the sequences of events in her daily routines extends to knowing not only the point in the day when she has her breakfast, but also that she is first placed in her highchair, then given her bib, then given her food – which is possibly presented in a predictable order – then the bib is removed, her hands are washed and she is lifted out of the highchair. This knowledge immensely supports her learning of new words, whose meanings she can associate with meanings of words previously learned in the course of her routines. The name of a new food, for example, would be learned in association with other foods during a meal, or when seen out shopping displayed alongside known foods.

At this stage, children recognize and identify a vast range of common objects and pictures of common objects when they are labelled (i.e. *nouns*) (Bzoch and League 1991); they also demonstrate an understanding of words other than names of objects, including action words (i.e. verbs), for example 'come', 'sit', 'drink', 'eat', 'walk'; and words used to refer to objects and people, without actually naming them (i.e. *pronouns*), for example 'you', 'me', 'mine'. During the couple of months leading up to her second birthday, the young child's understanding of more *complex sentences* starts to take off (Bzoch and League 1991). Her ability to follow sentences like 'I'll buy you some chocolate buttons when we go shopping' and 'Let's put your boots on because it's wet outside' involves some reasoning, world knowledge and some appreciation of time concepts in addition to understanding of the actual words used.

Communication and expressive skills in the second year: why do children communicate?

Language as an intellectual tool

When children start using language and learning names of objects, they are thought to reinforce their concepts of these objects by naming them as they handle them (Cooper *et al.* 1978). As they play, they make appropriate sounds (for example animal and vehicle noises). A bit later on children produce running commentaries as they play, which are considered to strengthen the ideas they are working out. During the second year, when children are just beginning to develop their language skills, they need to attend completely to whatever task they are currently engaged in, thus giving themselves the opportunity to consolidate the concepts they are exploring.

As their language skills become increasingly sophisticated over the forthcoming months and years, children use language increasingly to help them think, to make sense of their experiences, to regulate their behaviour, to develop their memory and modify their emotions (Hetherington and Parke 1986).

Social interaction

Interaction with carers continues to provide the major context for development of communication skills, including language. As in the later parts of the first year, young children in their second year communicate primarily for social reasons – that is, to engage in social interactions with someone else. The development of language is seen as serving the broader functions of regulating another's behaviour, engaging in social interaction and establishing joint attention (Westby 1998). Table 2.2 outlines the reasons for communicating (or 'communicative functions') that emerge between 10 and 18 months (Halliday 1975, cited by Westby 1998: 184). The functions which regulate another person's behaviour (requesting actions/ objects and protesting) are less socially motivated than the later emerging functions which (a) direct another person's attention to the child for social purposes (social interaction) and (b) direct another person's attention for the purposes of sharing the focus on an entity or event (joint attention) (Wetherby and Prizant 1993). Children may communicate for a wide range of reasons, and use both nonverbal and verbal skills. Over the second half of the second year, children begin to ask questions (mainly for information), make acknowledgments and give answers. Emergence of commenting on what cannot be seen – the first communicative function that relies on language for its expression – usually occurs around 24 months (Halliday 1975, cited by Westby 1998).

Early into the second year, the baby has established a sense of herself as separate from others (Hetherington and Parke 1986) and often initiates interaction using gestures, sounds or words. Around this time she will begin to test and tease adults (Reddy 1999) and may watch an adult's face for feedback when she is doing something she knows she is not supposed to do, to see how far she can go. She is able to ask adults for specific games or songs rather than for social contact in general.

The young child's interactions with other children also develop. At 1 year old she imitates other children in play and cooperates in simple play routines, such as rolling a ball or pushing a truck. A couple of months later she interacts with other children by touching, cuddling, pushing, hitting and taking toys away. She develops turn-taking sequences with another child which may start in a simple routine such as playing peekaboo and develop around 16 months into holding conversations, together with appropriate eye contact, gesture, focus of attention (such as a toy) and tuneful babble with the odd recognizable word.

Table 2.2 Communicative functions emerging between 10 and 18 months

Function	Examples
Regulating behaviour	
Request for object	Child points at beaker / vocalizes / says 'juice'
Request for action	Child raises arms up / says 'up'
Protest of actions	Mother wipes child's face / child cries / says 'no'
Rejection of object	Child throws unwanted doll to floor / says 'no doll'
Social interaction	
Gains attention of people in order to greet or initiate interaction	Child looks at / smiles at / tugs at mother / waves / says 'bye-bye' / calls out / says 'mama'
Expresses feelings or interest	Child smiles / cries / laughs / whines / says 'yum-yum', 'nice', 'yucky'
Requests social routines	Child holds hand out for parent to play 'Round and round the garden' / says 'Do roun roun'
Shows off to attract attention	Child puts on amusing facial expression / silly voice
Establishing joint attention	
Gives objects to people	Child gives mother a teddy / says 'here you are'
Shows objects to people	Child shows father her toes by pointing / says 'my tootsies'
Comments on objects	Child points at dog / says 'dog'
Comments on actions / events	Child points at cat eating / says 'he eating'
Requests information	Quizzical facial expression / rising intonation on vocalization / says 'What that?'
Comments on what cannot see	Child says 'Want yoghurt' when none is in sight

Source: Adapted from Westby (1998) with permission from Lippincott Williams & Wilkins.

Example 2.5 Communication to derive social pleasure

Soon after her first birthday Rowan started playing 'teaser'. The game involved offering an interesting toy or piece of food to her mother or father, coupled with an engaging smile. Just as her parent's hand reached out to take the offering, she would retract it quickly, with a satisfied giggle, soon joining in with her parents as they said, 'Teaser!'

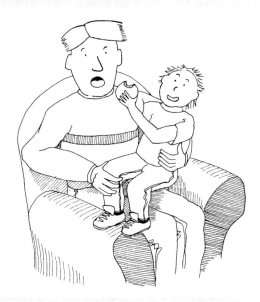

Figure 2.5 Twelve-month-old Rowan teasing her father with a biscuit

Despite a gradual increase in interest in other children, young children have a lot yet to learn about engaging peers in pleasurable social interaction (Garvey 1977) and will need to develop their communication skills in particular in order to become more socially versatile (see Examples 2.6 and 2.7).

Development of conversation skills in the second year

Young children wishing to engage in social interaction will do so most effectively by mastering the ambient language and learning the rules governing interaction. This is essentially what is involved in developing conversation skills. The communicative exchanges that started developing in the first year (mutual looking, smiling, back and forth vocalization, interactive games like peekaboo and pat-a-cake) are rule governed, like all communicative exchanges (Lees and Urwin 1991). Learning what is involved in these rules is to do with learning conversation skills.

Example 2.6 Interaction between peers – turn-taking and teasing

Both 15 months old, Rowan and her friend Ruby spontaneously started playing an interactive game with one another. Ruby was seated under a table with the tablecloth partially covering her face and body. She and Rowan were looking at each other when Ruby suddenly smiled. She then pulled the cloth in front of her face, hiding it completely. Rowan instantly recognized the game so tantalizingly initiated by Ruby, and they spent the next few minutes engaged in an entertaining round of peekaboo with each other.

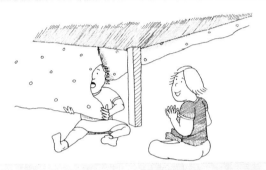

Figure 2.6 Rowan and Ruby playing peekaboo with each other at 15 months

Shortly after this game, Ruby was playing with a fun-sounding noisy toy. She looked at Rowan, whose eyes were fixed on the toy as Ruby waved it around. Ruby then held the toy out to Rowan, who in turn made eye contact with Ruby. As Rowan moved her hand towards the toy, Ruby smiled and, instead of relinquishing it as Rowan had clearly anticipated, she pulled it back, with the result that Rowan burst into howls of protest.

Turn-taking in the second year

The previous chapter describes a conversation as a series of turns, or communicative exchanges. Brinton and Fujiki (1989) cite Ninio and Bruner's study (1978) which concludes that mother and child turn-taking is highly efficient in book sharing activities in children aged 8 to 18 months. From 18 months, children can participate in conversations that involve each partner taking two turns (as in Example 2.8).

Many caregivers adopt ways of structuring communicative exchanges (or conversations) with their babies and young children to facilitate the development of conversational skills, notably turn-taking. Brinton and Fujiki (1989) also cite Schaffer, Collis and Parsons' (1977) study finding that 1- and 2-year-old children were able to engage in effective verbal turn-taking with minimal incidence of simultaneous speech. In summary, children up to the age of 2 have mastered the following about conversational turn-taking:

Example 2.7 Interaction between peers – taunting and talking

When they were 16 months old, Rowan and Grainne spent an afternoon together. For a good hour and a half they spent their time taking toys from each other, crying when the other had a toy, imitating each other pushing, sitting in and sitting on a trolley, and grappling for each other's food and beakers. They hit, poked, squeezed and tweaked each other throughout. Eventually they sat together on the bottom stair, held a short conversation then egged each other on to toddle off down the corridor to the front door and back to the stairs again.

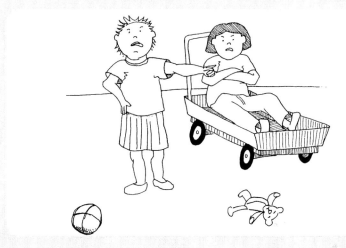

Figure 2.7 Rowan and Grainne taunt each other at 16 months

- turns alternate in conversation, and
- only one person talks at a time.

Two-year-olds are able to utilize this knowledge, but not in every communicative situation. Ervin-Tripp (1979), cited by Brinton and Fujuki (1989) found that at this age, children still allow long pauses in conversation and find it hard to break into other people's conversations due to difficulty in contributing something novel about an established *topic*. Pauses are believed to be particularly significant in acting as cues to 1- and 2-year-old children to take their turn in conversations.

Topic manipulation in the second year

The ability to manipulate topic in a conversation is a fundamental skill which Mogford and Bishop (1993a) describe in terms of:

- the ability to share a focus of attention (or topic of conversation)

Example 2.8 Conversational turn-taking between adult and child

At 18 months, Rowan and her mother had the following conversation involving two turns each. Rowan picked up her teddy and looked towards her mother.

ROWAN: Teddy.
MOTHER: That's your teddy.
ROWAN: *(making the teddy jump up)* Up.
        (looks at mother in anticipation)
MOTHER: Down *(as Rowan brings the teddy down again)*.

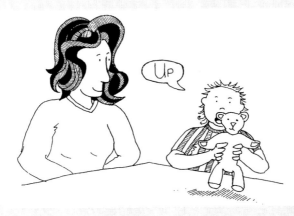

Figure 2.8 Eighteen-month-old Rowan and her mother take turns in a conversation

- the ability to recognize when there has been a change in the topic of conversation, and
- the ability to initiate a new topic of conversation, maintain it and develop it.

Topic manipulation is an aspect of conversational skills development that becomes more elaborate as children enter their second year and acquire increasingly more complex communication skills (Brinton and Fujuki 1989). Children of this age direct adults' attention to objects and events other than themselves through the use of gesture (for example pointing at a bird outside the window) and, later, words ('bird', 'look', 'baby', 'ball'). Foster (1981, 1986), cited by Brinton and Fujuki 1989, views this type of behaviour as the child initiating topics. The acquisition and use of words to direct another's attention elaborates the child's ability to initiate and expand topics triggered by immediate surroundings and increasingly from more abstract ideas. Parental support is highly significant in facilitating topic development in children of this age. The way parents respond to children's utterances is believed to support their developing abilities in initiating and maintaining topics in conversations.

Example 2.9 Developing the topic to keep the conversation going

At 19 months, Rowan and her father held the following conversation while looking at pictures in a book:

ROWAN: Piggy.
FATHER: That piggy's eating.
ROWAN: Eating.
FATHER: Piggy's eating bread.
ROWAN: Eating bread.
FATHER: And apples.

Rowan's father manages to construct a conversation with Rowan by expanding on her previous utterances. While Rowan initiated the topic of conversation, her father's expansions help them to maintain the topic.

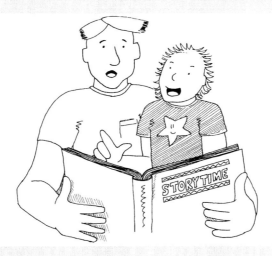

Figure 2.9 Rowan's father helps keep the conversation going with 19-month-old Rowan

As children's vocabulary and early grammatical development take off over the course of this and the subsequent year, so the likelihood of producing utterances topically linked to preceding adult utterances increases (Bloom, Rocissano and Hood 1976, in Brinton and Fujuki 1989).

Certain types of adult utterances have been noted as being more successful in influencing the ability to maintain topics in children of this age (Ervin-Tripp 1979, in Brinton and Fujuki 1989). Offering children choices is one way for adults to encourage children to keep talking about the same thing. The more a child is encouraged to maintain and develop a topic in conversation, the more opportunity they have to develop their language and communication skills. When adults talk about objects or events in which the child is currently engaged or showing an interest, they are in effect 'building a topical framework around the child's contribution' (Brinton and Fujuki 1989: 60). Similarly, repetitions or *expansions* of children's utterances serve to maintain topics the child has contributed to. Expansions involve the adult rephrasing the child's utterance and adding more words, which helps the child to learn more mature language structures. For example, the child says, 'doggy here' to which the adult responds, 'the doggy's running over here'.

Repairing conversations in the second year

Breakdowns in conversations are common, particularly in conversations involving young children. Recognizing when something has gone wrong with communication and developing ways of *repairing the conversation* is a skill which develops gradually but its beginnings can be seen in children between the ages of 1 and 2 (Brinton and Fujuki 1989). If she receives no response or not the desired response, the child repeats herself, alters her message or finds another way to convey her message. Additionally, she can respond to requests by other people to clarify her message. Observations of children's spontaneous self-repairs are evidence that children as young as 2 monitor the language they produce in the early stages of language production. Brinton and Fujuki speculate that repairs in children this young are rarely picked up by adult listeners for what they are unless they manifest as *dysfluent* speech. Self-repairs are thought to occur more frequently in those aspects of language which are in the process of acquisition and which are therefore less stable forms in a given child's repertoire.

Using early words

Having covered the reasons underlying why children in their second year communicate, attention is now turned to developments in expressive language in terms of what aspects of language they learn, and how much. It is helpful to clarify what constitutes a child's first words. Bloom (1993) and Haynes (1998) state that a true word must sound relatively similar on the different occasions it is used by a child, and must be used in a consistent way to refer to a particular object or event in the environment. Haynes cites Owens (1996), who additionally suggests that in order for a word to qualify as a true word it should resemble the adult pronunciation. A child who says 'bi' when unambiguously referring to a biscuit, for example, and who continues to use that word when talking about biscuits over successive occasions is meeting all the above criteria for true word production, even though she will need to continue modifying her representation of how the word sounds in order to eventually match the adult pronunciation. It is important to differentiate between strings of sounds children produce in babble, some of which might resemble (fortuitously) words from the ambient language, for example 'mama', 'dada', and the intentional use of consistent sound patterns to identify reliably particular objects or events over time. The child who produces 'dada' while banging a drum or splashing in the bath is not using that utterance as a true word, unlike the child who produces 'dada' consistently when she identifies her father (or, in an overextended use of the word's meaning, men in general).

12 to 18 months

Early single-word vocabulary: 0 to 50 words

For several months into the second year, the young child continues to produce jargon that will continue to be accompanied by gestures such as pointing. As in comprehension, true word production typically starts within a few context-bound routines such as making animal noises in a familiar game or consistently producing a specific sound to request an object or activity (Bates *et al*. in press). True naming of objects starts by 12 to 13 months in most children, but these very early expressive vocabularies are notoriously unstable and are likely to come and go from the child's repertoire until about 10 words have been established (Bates *et al*. in press). Many of her early words will overlap with continued use of vocalizations and gestures such as pointing for a few more months (Bzoch and League 1991).

The types of early words used by young children are generally names of people, objects and events in her immediate environment that are very familiar and of great interest to her, and words that express change or movement (Bloom 1993). Children often acquire simple phrases, for example 'here-you-are' and 'all-gone', that are chunked together and used as single words. Word types can be categorized as in Table 2.3, after Nelson 1973 (cited by Haynes 1998). Haynes (1998) emphasizes the variability among children regarding the age at which their vocabularies number 50 words; parental diaries record ages from 16 months to 22 months. Another key feature of the early word period is that the number of words they understand exceeds that of the number of words they use by an approximate ratio of 4:1 (Haynes 1998).

18 to 24 months

The vocabulary spurt

Many child language researchers have observed a rapid increase in the rate at which young children learn and use new words (see Bates *et al*. in press, Bloom 1993, Haynes 1998). Onset of the '*vocabulary spurt*' (Bloom 1993) occurs in most children between 14 and 20 months of age, and approximately 6 months after they have produced their first words. They start to use many more action words and other word types than previously. Relevance of cognitive developments to the vocabulary spurt is discussed by Bloom, who states:

> one cannot know the name for an object unless one also knows about objects;
> that they exist, are acted upon, and relate to each other and to themselves in
> more or less consistent ways
>
> (Bloom 1993: 100)

Table 2.3 Structure and content of an early vocabulary

Category	Words from Rowan's expressive vocabulary between 10 and 16 months[1]				
General names	**Food**	**Body**	**Care**	**Toys**	**General**
	banana	bottom	soap	ball	baby
	juice	toe	nappy	bubble	flower
	apple	fingers	bath	book	keys
	pear	ear	sponge	balloon	car
	broccoli	teeth	bib	pegs	music
	bread	nose	brush	doll	paper
	crisps	hands		trolley	
	cheese	eye	**Clothes**		**Containers**
	yoghurt	hair	boot	**Animals**	bag
	biscuit	knee	shoes	baabaa	box
	chocolate		jacket	duck	
	butter	**Utensils**	trousers	rabbit	**In the house**
	tea	fork	dress		chair
	porridge	spoon			door
		beaker			telly
Specific names	Cynthia	Anne	mummy	daddy	Po
	Teletubbies	teddy			
Action words	up	down	bounce	titty	poo
	woofwoof	gone	put/put it	bang	digging
Personal social	hello	byebye	boo	no	yes
	look	oops	ooh		
Modifiers	more	hot			
Function words	off	there	outside		

Note: 1 Rowan's pronunciations did not as yet match adult pronunciations, but were simplified
versions. Her use of some words also differed from adult meanings, hence the grouping of
some non-action words as actions.

She suggests that the quantitative increase in number of words used by children which characterizes the vocabulary spurt is indicative of qualitative changes occurring in their underlying thinking abilities. Haynes (1998) outlines changes evident in *constructional play* behaviours, object permanence and categorization ability around this stage in children's development. Bloom (1993) suggests that the vocabulary spurt occurs when children make the cognitive leap in understanding that everything has a name, and when they begin to appreciate the relations between words, or that words define other words. They begin to group words together, such as names of animals – cat, mouse, dog, pig, horse – and even to give a name to the category itself (in this case, 'animals'). The implication of words cueing other words thematically is that children, making connections between words, are poised to combine them to make simple phrases. Prior to using approximately fifty separate words, children's vocabularies are not thought to be organized according to the relations between words, but exist more as a group of separate, self-defining words. This notion links closely to what is suggested on pages 57–59 about children's conceptual and semantic development. Bates *et al.* (in press) observe a significant increase in the range of different types of words acquired over the course of the vocabulary spurt, with a proportional increase in the number of verbs, *adjectives* (descriptive words such as 'big', 'soft', 'short') and word types other than nouns.

It is highly tempting to suggest, as do Bates *et al.* (in press), and Bloom (1993), that these changes are indicative of a qualitative difference in the way word meanings are acquired, from the self-defining nature of object names (a cat or a teddy is always a cat or a teddy), to the relational meanings implicit in words other than nouns, such as 'big', 'hot', 'running'. These words require combination with other words in order for their meanings to be fully released, for example 'big teddy', 'hot milk', 'mummy running'. There may be startling differences between children of the same age in this period regarding the number of words used. While some at 20 months may be using ten words, other children's expressive vocabularies may extend to around fifty words (Bates *et al.* in press). In a further study undertaken by Dale, Bates, Reznick and Morrissett (1989), in Paul (1995), average vocabulary size at 20 months was 168 words.

Combining words

The onset of word combinations marks another important milestone in the acquisition of communication skills. Children usually start to combine two words together to make short phrases some time between their expressive vocabulary numbering 50 and 100 words, and typically between 18 and 20 months (Bates *et al.* in press). Once they have started to combine two words together, their expressive language development is at the *two-word level*. Again, there is a high level of variability regarding when children start to combine words, from as early as 14 months to some time into their second year. During the early stages of *two-word phrases*, the young child will continue to use many single words in addition to nonverbal ways of communicating. Before they spontaneously combine words, children go through a stage of imitating some two- and *three-word phrases* (Bzoch and League 1991).

Once children start spontaneously combining two or more words, we have evidence that they have started to make links between people, objects, actions and events that are part of their world. This crucial development is reflected in the early use of syntax, when children start to combine words according to certain rules rather than in a random manner (Tager-Flusberg 1989). Universally, children's early word combinations share certain characteristics (Tager-Flusberg 1989, Tomasello and Brooks 1999):

- Multiple words are uttered, which identify different participants of a scene or event, and which bear some relation to each other; for example, 'More biscuit' identifies the event of recurrence, and the biscuit itself.
- Some children may use a particular (favourite) word in combination with others. An example is the frequent combination of the word 'more' to identify recurrence of something, as in 'More juice', 'More biscuit', 'More tickle'.

- The order of words uttered generally conforms to a consistent pattern, as in the examples above 'more' occurs before the object word in each case.
- Word combinations are not repeated phrases that other people say; rather, they are novel utterances.
- Nouns, verbs and adjectives tend to dominate early word combinations, resulting in use of the term '*telegraphic speech*' for this stage.
- The content of early word combinations tends to focus on objects – their names, locations and attributes, who owns them and what is being done to them and by whom. The interrelationships between objects, people and actions provide a focus for young children's thoughts and verbal expressions universally.

Twenty-month-old children all around the world encode the same basic group of relational meanings in their early word combinations (Bates *et al.* in press), which are listed below:

- existence – appearance, disappearance, reappearance of interesting objects or events
- desires – refusal, denial, requests
- basic event relations – agent–action–object, possession, change of state or change of location
- attribution – 'hot', 'pretty' and so on.

See Table 2.4 for examples of early word combinations and relational meanings that they encode. As with single words, the same combinations of words can be used to express a range of meanings. The phrase 'Phoebe bed' might be used to express 'That's Phoebe's bed'; 'Where is Phoebe's bed?' or 'Phoebe is in bed'. Once again, intonation, gesture, body language and the context in which the phrase is uttered help towards deducing the child's intended meaning. While the order of words uttered may not match that of the adult language initially, it does so in a short time.

Table 2.4 Early word combinations produced by Phoebe at 24 months

Word combination	Intended meaning	Relational meaning
daddy gone	daddy has gone	existence–disappearance
want biscuit	I want a biscuit	desire–request
bye-bye train	the train has gone	existence–disappearance
more juice	I want more juice	desire–request
Phoebe bed	that's Phoebe's bed	possession
allgone cake	I've finished my cake	existence–disappearance
mummy there	mummy's in there	location
Jojo teddy	that's Jojo's teddy	possession
duck gone	the duck's gone	existence–disappearance

Early grammatical development

The start of word combinations and cognitive developments in areas such as memory mean that the young child is soon able to talk beyond what is happening in her immediate environment at the current time (the 'here and now'), to include past and possibly future events. She will continue to supplement her words with some jargon, gestures and acting out. She will soon start to use *negative* forms by using the words 'No' or 'Not' at the beginning of phrases, for example 'No biscuit' might express 'I don't want a biscuit' or 'There aren't any biscuits'. She will notably start to ask questions that require a 'Yes' or 'No' answer, signalled in the early stages by a questioning intonation on utterances such as 'Rowan drink?' meaning, 'Is that Rowan's drink?' A little later she will start to use 'Where' and 'What' at the start of questions, as in 'Where's mummy?' and 'What's that?' (Tager-Flusberg 1989). In addition to using negatives and early question forms, the child approaching 2 may start to use pronouns, generally in the following order (Chiat 1986):

1 I, me, mine
2 it
3 you, your.

They soon start to refer to themselves by name. As children's vocabularies increase in the range and quantity of words used, so they are able to make a wider range of word combinations and start to develop grammar. Towards the end of this year, the young child may start to imitate some three-word phrases as a precursor to spontaneously producing three-word phrases herself, generally with very clear meanings, for example, 'Mummy drink milk', 'Roro want more'.

Early speech

The sounds that occur in children's earliest words are closely linked to the sounds that predominated in their babbling during the previous months. Towards the end of the first year, babbling develops into more varied patterns of consonant–vowel combinations (jargon). With this development come some recognizable early words and word approximations (Stackhouse and Wells 1997).

Most children's early speech attempts share certain characteristics. After the onset of early words, it usually takes until a child is 4½ or sometimes later before they can accurately pronounce all the sounds of English in words (Grunwell 1987). As early words emerge, sounds and words are simple, usually consisting of only a consonant and a vowel, or with the consonant and vowel repeated, for example 'mama', 'dada', 'byebye', 'no', 'yumyum'.

Early sound simplification patterns

Children at this stage simplify the pronunciation of words they find hard to say by using systematic *simplification patterns* where parts of words or some sounds may be omitted, or easier sounds may be used in place of more difficult ones. Stackhouse and Wells (1997) observe that the simplification processes that tend to be applied at this stage are those that affect the shape of the whole word, rather than individual sounds. So, initial syllables might be duplicated (*initial syllable reduplication*), two or more consonants might be pronounced as a single consonant (*consonant harmony*), all consonants occurring at beginning of words might be pronounced with activation of the vocal folds to produce voice (*context sensitive voicing*, for example voicing of the initial sound – see pages 6–8 for more detail on voicing), whole syllables might be deleted (*weak syllable deletion*), or final consonants might always be deleted (*final consonant deletion*). Sound *blends* are reduced to just one sound (*blend reduction*). Examples of these simplification processes can be found in Table 2.5.

Table 2.5 Examples of systematic simplification processes applied in early speech (Rowan at 16 months)

Target word	Rowan's pronunciation	Type of simplification process
dolly	dodo	initial syllable reduplication
tiger	giger	consonant harmony
tea	dea	context sensitive voicing
yoghurt	yog	weak syllable deletion
bath	ba	final consonant deletion
dress	des	blend reduction

When several simplifications occur together, as is usually the case at this stage of development, it can be very hard to work out what children are saying. While these patterns are common among children, each child will differ in their use of simplifications.

Why do children use simplification patterns?

Explaining phonological development (which includes knowing how to use speech sounds meaningfully) has posed a challenge to child language researchers over the years. The transition from *prelinguistic* sound production where a vast range of sounds might be produced, to the systematic use of sounds according to a rule governed system (a phonological system) whereby children's pronunciations of words conform to those of the ambient language involves a major learning process, coupled with necessary developments in motor skills and speech processing. Essentially, children have to learn that sounds of a language are used contrastively to convey differences in meaning among words. Until a child is aware of this fact, she may see no reason to alter her pronunciation and continue to pronounce the words 'did', 'stick', 'tick', 'dig', 'sick', and 'sit' all as 'did'. Such a child's speech would be very difficult to understand, in particular if her speech production skills did not develop in line with her increasing vocabulary and grammatical skills. Younger children are, however, constrained in the range and type of sounds they are able to produce accurately (if adult pronunciation is taken as the standard), due to immaturities in motor control and physical developments of the speech musculature. Mature pronunciation of speech sounds in connected speech involves an extremely high level of motor control, speech being the most complex of all motor activities (Borden and Harris 1984, Grunwell 1987, Hewlett 1990, Love and Webb 1992). The application of simplification patterns in child speech is seen by some researchers (Hewlett 1990) as a means of simplifying articulation of sounds and words that are difficult to pronounce, *while being able to perceive* the discrepancies between their own and others' pronunciations. As a child's articulatory skill develops, her need to apply simplification patterns reduces. Her phonological system thus undergoes a series of successive reorganizations on the way to achievement of mature pronunciation patterns.

Common early sounds

The group of sounds that children commonly use in their early words include 'm', 'p', 'b', 'w', 'n', 't', and 'd', in addition to vowels. Of course there will be variation among children, but these sounds are expected to emerge during the second year (Grunwell 1987). Some children will be using sounds such as 'k', 'g' and 's'. There is quite a lot of evidence to suggest that children's early words are partly influenced by the sounds they favour, which are restricted at first. At 14 months, Rowan's expressive vocabulary consisted largely of words with the sound 'd' in them (duck, down, dolly, teddy, daddy). Additionally, she pronounced many other sounds in words as 'd' (baby → daydy; juice → doos; bye-bye → duh-dye). By 16 months, however, 21 per cent of her words started with the sound 'b'. Young children early on may avoid words containing sounds not part of his or her favoured range (Menn 1989). With the vocabulary spurt that occurs around 20 months, the range of sounds used increases. Use of babble (or 'jargon') continues as early words develop but will gradually fade out by the start of the third year.

Achieving consistent pronunciations of words

Physical factors such as maturation of the nervous system and muscle coordination contribute to how sounds and words are made in the early stages of speech development. Research suggests that at this stage children store words as whole units in their memories, unlike at later stages when other factors come into play which enable segmentation of words into smaller units such as syllables and sounds (Stackhouse and Wells 1997). As the number of words and sounds in a child's expressive vocabulary increases, the ways words are pronounced become more variable in these early days. This variability is related to the child's difficulty in coordinating fine muscular movements in a consistent way. 'More' was one of Rowan's earliest words – she used it frequently but did not stabilize her pronunciation for several months. Her pronunciations included: 'mer', 'mmm', 'ma', 'mar', 'muh', 'mo' and 'more'.

Pronunciations become more consistent as the young child develops better muscle coordination. Children need to hear a word repeated many times in order to build up their perceptual and productive knowledge of it. How children perceive words is thought to be as important in influencing pronunciation, especially in this early stage, as their articulatory abilities.

Intonation

By the end of the second year, English-speaking children have mastered the features of intonation necessary to signal the difference between an utterance consisting of a series of single words, 'look', 'daddy', and a phrase consisting of two or more words, 'look daddy' (Crystal 1986). Whereas in single-word utterances, each word is made with equal, or nearly equal *stress*, two-word utterances that start to occur around 18 months come to be produced within a discrete intonation contour with appropriate emphasis, or contrastive stress on one syllable, depending on the intended meaning. Children have worked out which syllable requires emphasis, or stress, and the use of loudness to signal stress is not random. In the utterance 'look *da*ddy' (where the italicized syllable signals the stressed syllable, or syllable which is spoken with most loudness) the listener is informed that 'daddy' is the most important piece of information in the utterance, and that he or she should look at him. In the utterance '*look* daddy', the listener is 'daddy' and he is being requested to look at something that has caught his child's attention. Another feature which signals multi-word phrases as opposed to a series of single words is that intervening pauses between the words comprising phrases become less likely in subsequent repetitions. The earliest questions children ask are formed by using rising pitch of voice on two-word combinations, as in 'Mummy here?', 'Daddy gone?', 'My teddy?' Accurate interpretation of the meanings of these phrases is determined by factors within the context and the phrase itself.

Summary of Chapter 2

Attention and learning language

1   Children's attention is single-channelled, making it hard for them to attend simultaneously to two sources of information (for example visual and verbal).

Play and symbolic understanding

2   Pretend play, which is thought to be closely linked to language development, emerges early in the second year and gradually increases in complexity with development.

Understanding meaning

3 Children's understanding of word meanings is gradual and is affected by the context in which the word is spoken.

4 It is necessary for a child to learn first the concepts of objects, actions, people and events before she can begin to understand the words that refer to them.

5 Children make errors in how they use early words, which are related to the nature of the underlying concepts they have for words, and to limited vocabulary.

Early verbal understanding

6 True verbal understanding of words is preceded by situational understanding of phrases, then situational understanding of words within phrases.

7 By the end of the second year, children can identify a wide range of objects and actions by their verbal labels; follow sentences containing two or three key words; and follow sentences involving a range of vocabulary, concepts and world knowledge.

Communication and expressive skills in the second year: why do children communicate?

8 Over the second year, children use their communication skills in various ways to engage in social interaction with others, to establish joint attention with others and to regulate the behaviour of others. As language emerges, its role as an aid to children's thinking and concept development becomes evident.

9 While children in the second year are interested in peers, they need to become more skilled communicators in order to engage in mutually enjoyable, sustained interactions.

10 Over the course of the second year, children have started to develop many conversational skills:

- the ability to signal an intention to communicate to a conversational partner in a way that they will recognize
- the ability to respond reciprocally to a partner's communication signals
- the ability to be both listener and speaker, or message recipient and transmitter
- the ability to take turns
- topic manipulation
- the ability to recognize when communication has gone wrong and to develop ways of repairing the conversation.

Using early words

11   First words are commonly produced in combination with gestures; use of
gestures subsides as verbal capacities increase.
12   Two-word phrases emerge after the vocabulary spurt, usually during the second
half of the year. By second birthdays, expressive vocabulary may range
between 50 and 200 words; children use some verbs and adjectives – however,
names of people and objects still predominate; they have started to apply
consistent rules when combining words, in particular with regards to word
order.

Early speech

13   Sounds used in later babbling are frequently among those favoured in early
words; children simplify pronunciations of words using systematic patterns
largely affecting the shape of the word at this stage.

Key skills 2.1 Communication skills usually achieved by 18-month-old
children

- Communicates primarily for social reasons
- Perseveres in conveying her message if it is not understood, by repeating or
  altering it
- Attracts people's attention by looking at them and pointing at an object or
  event
- Focuses on self-directed activities and attention is single-channelled
- Understands simple commands, questions and gestures (for example 'come
  here', 'give to mummy')
- Understands several new words each week
- Uses five to twenty words one at a time
- Names familiar objects and actions in everyday situations
- Uses the same word for different reasons (for example 'cat' could mean 'Is
  that a cat?', 'There's a cat' or 'Give me the cat')
- May use one word to talk about things that are linked in some way (for
  example 'apple' for apple, orange and peach), or restrict word meanings (for
  example 'apple' refers only to her apple that she has at dinner time, not to
  other apples)
- Intersperses real words in her babble (for example 'mamubaba-doggy-dada')

Before using this table, see page xxi.

Key skills 2.2 Communication skills usually achieved by 2-year-old children

- Communicates using a combination of gestures, looking, sounds and words
- Starts to take turns in conversations
- Able to attend to activity of own choosing
- Understands that events are made up of a series of steps in sequence (for example wash hands, sit at table, eat, get down)
- Demonstrates more than one action in pretend play (for example feeds doll then puts doll to bed)
- Understands that words can stand for pictures and toys of real objects
- Understands some long and complicated sentences
- Able to carry out instructions containing two key words, without contextual cues (for example 'Put teddy on the table')
- Starts to combine two or three words into short phrases (for example 'Mummy here', 'Teddy jump here')
- Uses the same word or phrase for different reasons (for example, 'Daddy drink' might mean, 'That's daddy's drink', 'Daddy, I want your drink' or 'Daddy's drinking')
- Starts to ask questions
- Starts to say 'No' and 'Not'
- Starts to talk about past events and possibly things that might happen in the future

---

Before using this table, see page xxi.

Warning signs 2.1 Possible warning signs for 18-month-old children

- **Shows little interest in what is going on around her**
- **Not developing appropriate relationships with others (for example, poor eye contact, lots of screaming, dislike of body contact)**
- **Showing little interest in playing with main carers and not demanding of their attention**
- **Uninterested in pushing and pulling toys and noisemakers**
- **Does not look round to see where sounds are coming from**
- **Does not respond to name being spoken**
- **Does not respond to familiar songs and rhymes**
- **Appears unable to follow short sentences like 'Let's find your coat'**
- **Little variety of speech sounds, babbling and no real words used**
- **Parents express concerns, are worried or anxious**

⚠ Before using this table, see page xxii.

Warning signs 2.2 Possible warning signs for 2-year-old children

- **Shows little interest in what is going on around her**
- **More difficult to control that would be expected**
- **Does not concentrate for short, intense periods on a self-chosen toy or activity**
- **Not showing signs of wanting to join in other children's play**
- **Does not want to help carers in their activities**
- **Does not begin to imitate actions in play (for example putting doll to bed, brushing hair, feeding doll)**
- **Not able to follow simple instructions in daily routine without gesture. May rely on copying others**
- **Does not understand the names of several everyday objects such as cup, spoon, shoe and biscuit**
- **Few clear single words used; no babbling or sentence-like utterances**
- **Stammering**
- **Not joining two words together**
- **Parents express concerns, are anxious or worried**

⚠ Before using this table, see page xxii.

The third year 3

Attention control

Over the course of the third year, children's control over their own focus of attention becomes gradually more flexible (Reynell 1980), but is still predominantly single-channelled as in the preceding year. It is still difficult for children to listen and respond appropriately to verbal directions if they are focused on an absorbing activity. It is often necessary for adults to help children at this stage to shift attention from the activity they are engaged in by first gaining their attention before giving them a verbal instruction. They might do this by calling the child's name, or saying 'Look'. Children at this stage are more receptive than previously in shifting attention from an activity to verbal directions and back to the activity, but need adult help. They still need to apply full auditory and visual attention to the speaker in order to carry out directions.

Implications of children's attention control at this stage for learning language are similar to those for children at the previous level as outlined in Chapter 2, 'Attention and learning language' (page 50). Language is more likely to be attended to, and thus learned, if it is introduced by the adult in ways which do not require the child to redirect their focus of attention and which are integral to the activity or focus of interest the child is currently attending to.

Example 3.1 Single-channelled attention

In her third year, Rowan frequently became absorbed in tidying up – this activity was as integral to the process and activity of play as others. On one occasion she was carefully replacing puzzle pieces in a tin after completing the puzzle when her mother, who was sitting behind her, tried unsuccessfully to attract her attention in order to give her some sweets. She called, 'Rowan, your chocolate buttons. Chocolate, chocolate buttons. Don't you want your chocolate buttons?' It was not until all the puzzle pieces were back in their tin that Rowan was ready to turn to her mother and say 'What?' On other occasions, when Rowan's attention was not fixed on an activity of her own choosing, she responded immediately to such offers! Chocolate buttons were always highly motivating, providing attention was not elsewhere.

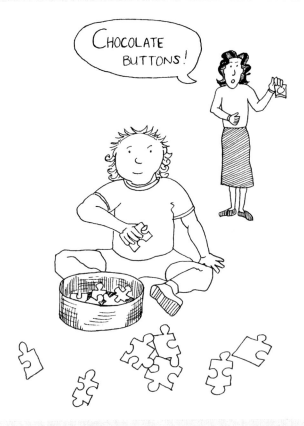

Figure 3.1 Rowan displaying single-channelled attention at 2½

Links between play and language

Children's play skills continue to expand and develop over the course of the third year. Broadly, the functions of play over this year are:

- to assist in children's cognitive development
- to advance their social development, especially through fantasy and role play
- to assist children in exploring their emotions.

It is possible to draw links between many different types of play and language skills development, but those aspects of play which are considered to be more important for language development will be considered here – imaginative play, including *symbolic play*, and role play. In the following sections, there is a description of relevant play behaviours with examples, a discussion on the role of language in play, and the relationship that exists between language development and play development.

Symbolic and imaginative play

Imaginative play is linked so closely to language development because it involves the child's ability to recognize and use symbols (Cooke and Williams 1985), without which verbal understanding cannot proceed.

Children start to extend the pretend play sequences which they started to develop towards the end of the preceding year (see Table 2.1, page 53) by not only having objects representing or standing in for real ones, but also by creating imaginary objects without props and attributing imaginary or representational objects with pretend properties (Harris 1989). The objects that are used in symbolic play might bear little perceptual similarity to those they represent.

The decrease in similarity of objects used by children in symbolic play to the things they represent leads on to the emergence of imaginary friends and other imaginary things such as sweets in pockets. This development occurs over the time that language development really takes off, during the third and later years. From the end of the second year onwards children require ever decreasing contextual support to understand the words and sentences that are spoken around them.

Children's developing sense of self coupled with the capacity for pretence enables them to start to understand and feel the needs and feelings of others (Harris 1989). Children start to re-enact recently experienced events and recombine them in new ways to create stories in which they might imagine they are other people and act out events which they might not have directly observed or experienced.

During the early part of the third year, dolls are endowed with the capacity for action and experience and are made to talk by children during play and to act out their wishes, needs and feelings (Harris 1989).

Cooper *et al.* (1978) discuss the role of children's verbal commentaries which accompany their play, drawing on the ideas of the twentieth century

Example 3.2 Use of objects in symbolic play

At 30 months, Rowan picked up a large plastic jug she found in the garden. She started putting handfuls of gravel in the jug.

ADULT: What have you got in there, Rowan?
ROWAN: Very hot, very hot. Got strawberries in it. *(Rowan places the jug on a brick on the ground)*
ROWAN: Very hot. Mustn't touch. Mustn't burn your fingers.
ADULT: Are you cooking?
ROWAN: Yes. I cooking uh strawberries.

Rowan's use of gravel to represent strawberries is truly symbolic. She takes another leap to make believe they are hot and therefore must not be touched.

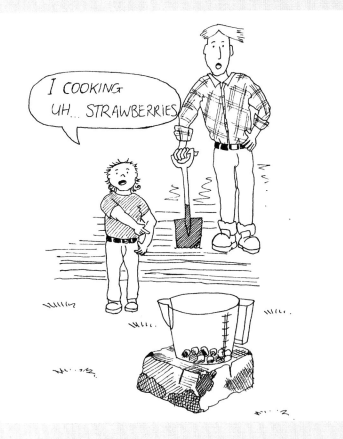

Figure 3.2 Rowan pretending to cook strawberries at 2½

Example 3.3 Increasing flexibility of objects in symbolic play

During her third year, Rowan frequently approached adults to show them new uses of objects that she had created:

- She put a clothes peg on the end of her finger and said, 'Look mum, crocodile!'
- She carefully arranged several glass beads inside the pages of a book, saying, 'This is my book. It's a mirror go inside. No, it's a present book.' As a few glass beads fell off, Rowan said, 'Oh. It fall off. It my raisin.'
- She held one end of a tie, allowing the other end to trail down the stairs, saying, 'It my snakey, mum. Snakey!' She repeated this afterwards using a pipe, then a pole.

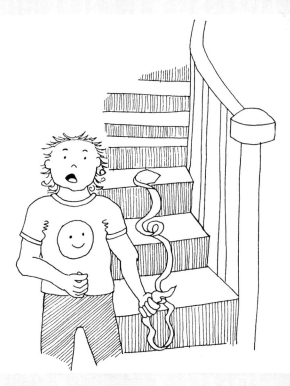

Figure 3.3 Rowan pretending that her dad's tie is her snake

- She placed one stacking ring on top of another, held them up to her eye and looked through them, saying 'It my camera.' She then adopted a still, smiling pose as her father took her 'picture'.

Example 3.4 Re-enacting recent experiences in pretend play

During the course of her third year, Rowan extended her pretend play sequences with her dolls to play different roles and develop stories that often drew on recent experiences. Following a short illness, she was playing with one of her dolls. She tucked the doll up in a make-believe bed and adopted a solicitous tone to say, 'You all right? You feeling better? Have your medicine now. Make you feel better.' A little later, Rowan announced, 'She my baby sister', and bundled her up in the toy pushchair to take her shopping.

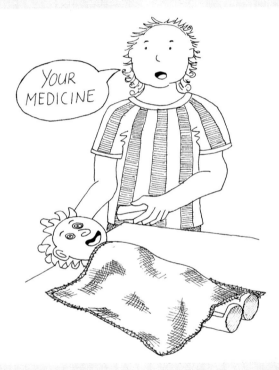

Figure 3.4 Rowan giving her doll some medicine, aged 2¾

neuropsychologist Luria (1961). At previous stages, children are thought to stabilize their concepts of the objects they label as they come across them in play. With the addition of a verbal commentary such as the one produced by Rowan in Example 3.5, children are thought to be consolidating the ideas they are currently working on through their play. There is a different dimension now to language as it is used by children to integrate different aspects of their activities.

In the second half of the third year, children enact less familiar events in their play, such as a visit to the zoo. Development of this type of play is supported by giving

Example 3.5 Dolls are endowed with human qualities and experiences

At 26 months, Rowan was playing with miniature dolls, cutlery and furniture. She produced the following commentary as she played: 'She's want sit on uh carpet.' The doll was made to sit on the carpet and Rowan started to give it food. 'Want it all? She's want more.' Rowan proceeded to use a spoon to mix imaginary food on a plate, which she then fed to the doll. 'Aah' she said, then smacked her lips. 'All gone. Now she's want some medicine.' Rowan lifts a cup to the doll's lips. 'Little bit. All gone.' Rowan then placed all the toys on a nearby shelf, saying as she did so, 'I put them up there. I put dolly up there. She's have enough.' Rowan's language skills clearly facilitate her to express the doll's actions and perceived wishes and internal states as they occur in her play.

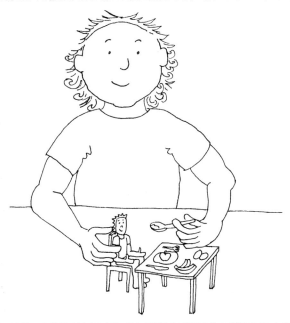

Figure 3.5 Rowan plays with miniature dolls, aged 26 months

children lots of different experiences which they will then want to talk about in their play, thus giving the opportunity for language development (Cooke and Williams 1985). As children act out in ever increasing detail events in their play which draw from their own observations and experiences, their understanding of the world grows. Talk with caregivers during this type of play encourages their understanding of the sequences of events and reinforces events, thus building up the child's memory and vocabulary.

Imaginative play develops over the year from the solitary symbolic activities which occur around the child's second birthday to become the complex, co-operative, make-believe play of the 3-year-old (Hetherington and Parke 1986). The fanciful, exaggerated pantomime of play that is seen in 3-year-olds enables them to try out future roles, experience the feelings and roles of others and function in a group with peers. For further information and discussion on the functions of play and the range of different play behaviours, please refer to Jeffree *et al.* (1985), Cohen (1993) and Bruner *et al.* (1985).

Role play and social play

Over the third year, there is a gradual increase in the amount of time children spend playing with other children, and a gradual decrease in the amount of time they spend playing with caregivers (Eckerman, Whatley and Kutz 1975, cited by Hetherington and Parke 1986). At this stage they play equally happily with opposite and same sex peers and experiment with reciprocal role relationships, such as being alternatively 'chaser' and 'chased', or 'hider' and 'seeker'. One of the key differences between playing with peers and caregivers is that caregivers facilitate sustained interaction during play while peers present more of a challenge to a child wishing to initiate interaction and maintain it. The more equal nature of peer interaction provides opportunities for children to try out the communication skills that they have been supported to develop with their more facilitative caregivers.

Towards the middle of the third year children will play with peers nearby, but do not as yet understand about sharing toys or adult attention. They may show strong interest in watching peers at play and will occasionally join in; it is not until the latter end of the year that they become actively involved in sustained make-believe play with peers, however (Sheridan 1997). Once children are fully involved in play with peers, play becomes a social activity in itself.

Social play allows children to observe and imitate others and provides a forum for extending communication skills (Cooke and Williams 1985). Children can be given opportunities to become more sociable and develop more confidence as communicators. There are lots of opportunities for extending cognitive, social and language skills in role play with peers which allows children to swap roles and thus explore a wider range of real and imaginary roles and scenarios.

Conceptual, semantic and vocabulary development

Vocabulary growth

Between the ages of 2½ and 4½, children acquire on average between two and four new words daily (Myers Pease *et al.* 1989). One of the most significant factors influencing the size of children's vocabularies at these stages is the language that they hear from adults in the environment. Hart and Risley (1995) cited by Weitzman

(1998) found average expressive vocabulary size (that is, the number of words children use, as opposed to the number of words they understand) for different groups of North American children at 30 months to vary between 357 and 766 words. Over the six month period leading up to their third birthdays, the different groups of children increased the size of their vocabulary by an average of 168 words and 350 words respectively. The difference in adult language input between the two groups was that parents of children with the larger vocabularies:

- talked significantly more to their children, thus using a wider vocabulary themselves
- asked more questions
- gave more positive feedback to what their children said
- prompted their children to take more turns
- managed to keep the conversation going for longer.

Parents of children with the smaller vocabularies:

- talked significantly less to their children, thus exposed them to narrower vocabularies
- had shorter conversations with their children.

Word categories

Myers Pease *et al.* (1989) discuss how strategies used by mothers when teaching children words give information on the hierarchical nature of words and their groupings. When teaching group members such as 'tractor', 'bus', 'train', they might point and give the object's name. When teaching the group name, they tend to say things like 'A car and a bus and a train. All of them are kinds of vehicles.' This type of explicit teaching may assist children in how they mentally categorize things in the world (Figure 3.6). This type of information, which is to do with how words define other words, is particularly useful for word learning at this and subsequent stages of language development.

Words for basic concepts

Learning words that relate to a range of basic concepts and which include adjectives (including 'hot', 'cold', 'thick', 'thin', 'big', 'small', 'red', 'blue') and *prepositions* ('in', 'on', 'under', 'behind', 'in front') starts during this year (Boehm 1976). By the time they are 3, children have developed an understanding of the following spatial terms (Boehm 1989, in Paul 1995: 295): 'in', 'in front of', 'beside', 'on', 'over', 'next to', 'out', 'under'. Myers Pease *et al.* (1989) report how learning of adjective pairs, such as 'hot' and 'cold' which have a polar relationship, generally involves learning the positive pair member first, followed some time later by the negative pair member. Overuse of one adjective to talk about both extremes of a

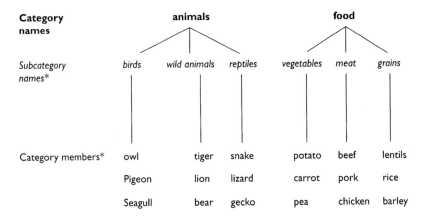

*There is a restricted set of examples given here, due to space limitations

Figure 3.6 Examples of categorical grouping of words in the mind

continuum, such as 'hot' for things that are both hot and cold, is not uncommon at this stage (see Example 3.6).

Order of acquisition of the words 'in', 'on', 'under' was found by Clark (1973), cited by Myers Pease *et al.* (1989), to be related closely to how children act on objects. They have a natural tendency to put things in other things, such as buttons in boxes and spoons in cups, before they put things on or under other things. These behaviours seem to have a bearing on children's conceptual development, which in turn influences the rate at which they understand words relating to concepts, and how they respond to instructions involving these words (see 'The probable location strategy', page 94).

Myers Pease *et al.* (1989) discuss findings from a range of studies looking at how children acquire colour names. Relevant factors include:

- perceptual saliency
- adult teaching which involves providing relevant conceptual information
- possibly a unique pattern of acquisition for colours pertaining to a predisposition to take particular notice of the field of colour.

During their third year, children are often able to name two or three colours.

Understanding words and sentences

As outlined in previous sections of the book, comprehension involves a lot more than being able to understand the words that are spoken in a sentence. In real communicative situations, children comprehend what is spoken to them by making use of:

Example 3.6 Understanding and using words for an opposite pair

Before Rowan learned to use the word 'hot', she signalled that something was hot by taking a sharp intake of breath with her lips rounded, in the way her parents had done to warn her not to touch hot things like mugs of tea and radiators. She then started to use the word 'hot' appropriately for many hot things, and soon afterwards started using 'cold' when she put her fingers in cold water. It appeared that she had sorted out the relative meanings of the two words. After a couple of weeks or so, however, she started mixing up her use of 'hot' and 'cold' to refer indiscriminately to hot, warm and cold things. It took a few more weeks before she was reliable in her use of the words hot and cold.

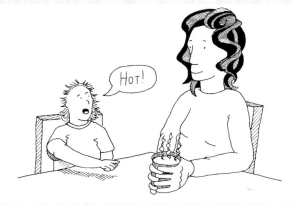

Figure 3.7 Two and a half-year-old Rowan describing a mug of tea as 'hot'

A tentative explanation for Rowan's pattern of learning is presented below:

1 Rowan first learned about the positive extreme of the concept hot, and used the word appropriately in a number of contexts.
2 Rowan then learned to use the word cold, but she restricted her use of this word at first to one context, suggesting that she had not learned the underlying concept.
3 As Rowan's conceptual understanding developed, she needed to reorganize her understanding of 'hot' and 'cold', placing them in polar relation to one another along the same dimension of temperature. This process of conceptual reorganization was reflected at this time in her confused use of the words 'hot' and 'cold'.
4 Rowan arrived at a more mature understanding of the concept of temperature as a dimension with extreme values at either end, which can be referred to by using the words 'hot' and 'cold'.

- knowledge they have about what usually happens in different situations
- contextual information in the form of objects and events in the immediate environment that provide additional support to understanding any language that is spoken
- nonverbal information carried in the speaker's facial expression, tone of voice, gestures, body language and position
- their understanding of words and sentences spoken.

Comprehension strategies used in the third year

Children between the ages of 2 and 3 make use of a range of strategies to assist their comprehension. These strategies will change as children develop.

The probable event strategy

During the third year, children can process sentences involving three separate pieces of information which comply with expectations about certain events, such as 'Mummy feeds the baby'; 'The dog chases the cat'; 'Daddy pats the dog', and will be able to carry out relevant instructions using toys (Chapman 1978 in Paul 1995). If asked to carry out instructions using the same set of toys but reversing their roles within the sentences and thus describing less probable events, as in 'The baby feeds mummy'; 'The cat chases the dog'; 'The dog pats daddy', children will still select the appropriate toys for each instruction from a selection but will interpret the instructions in the more probable direction. This means they will make the mummy feed the baby in response to both instructions 'Make the mummy feed the baby' and 'Make the baby feed the mummy'.

The probable location strategy

Children at this stage respond to instructions involving placing objects in or on others using their knowledge about where those objects are usually placed (Chapman 1978, in Paul 1995). For example, a child should respond appropriately to instructions such as 'Put the spoon in the cup'; 'Put the knife on the plate'; but might not place objects correctly in response to instructions such as 'Put the spoon on the cup'; 'Put the knife in the cup'.

Supplying missing information

Children at this stage demonstrate that they know that questions asked of them require responses and will supply answers even though they have not fully understood the question (James 1990, in Paul 1995).

Developments in verbal understanding between 24 and 30 months

This section is concerned with the words and word combinations that children understand. Children's *receptive vocabularies* are expanding rapidly and they are able to recognize the names and pictures of most common objects. They can identify objects from functional definitions as in 'Which one do we cook with/eat with/ wash with?', and point to smaller parts of the body such as chin, elbow, eyebrow (Bzoch and League 1991). They respond appropriately to questions that start with 'What . . .?' and 'Where . . .?' (James 1990, in Paul 1995). Their conceptual development assists them to recognize a greater number of categories, including knowing that family members have names like 'grandma', 'uncle' and 'sister' (Bzoch and League 1991). Although they still make use of comprehension strategies and nonlinguistic cues, children at this stage are far less reliant on nonlinguistic information in order to make sense of what others say.

Developments in verbal understanding between 30 and 36 months

During the second half of the third year, children demonstrate an understanding of all familiar object names, of all common action words and of most common adjectives (Bzoch and League 1991). They respond appropriately to questions that start with 'Who . . .?', 'Whose . . .?', 'Why . . .?' and occasionally 'How many . . .?' (James 1990, in Paul 1995). By the time most children are 3 they are able to process and follow sentences involving three separate pieces of information, or three key words (Bzoch and League 1991), such as 'Give the *big book* to *grandma*'; '*Mummy* and *Joe* are going to the *park*'; 'Get *Daddy's hat* from the *cupboard*'. This is sometimes referred to as the '*three-word stage*'.

The wealth of knowledge that 3-year-olds have acquired about concrete things in their environment like people, animals, food, toys, vehicles, clothes, buildings and places, in addition to more abstract knowledge such as feelings, sequencing of events and simple causal relationships means that they are able to follow a wide range of stories that relate to their everyday lives.

Communication and expressive skills in the third year

Social and cognitive developments influencing communication and language development

Social and cognitive developments over the course of this year enable children to start taking listeners' perspectives into account during interaction. One way this is illustrated is through the gradual move towards correct use of terms such as 'there', 'here', 'go', 'come', 'I', and 'you', which necessarily requires distinguishing the perspectives of the self as speaker from that of the listener (Pan and Snow 1999). Children's developing sense of self during this period facilitates correct use of pronouns 'I' and 'you', which involves seeing the self as an object and taking another's perspective towards one's self (Maccoby 1980).

As young as 3, some children were found by Bates (1976, cited by Pan and Snow 1999) to increase the number of politeness markers (for example 'please') to requests addressed to older or less familiar listeners, thus demonstrating the ability to take these listeners' perspectives into account. Two-year-olds were found by Dunn and Kendrick, cited by Warren-Leubecker and Bohannon (1989) to talk differently when addressing younger siblings to when they address adults. Adapting communication for younger listeners might involve using a higher pitch voice, shorter phrases and a greater number of commands. Children might also adapt their communication in this way when addressing animals and their dolls.

Another way in which children demonstrate an ability to shift perspective from their own is through their use of language in fantasy and role play (Example 3.7).

The development of conversation skills

Keeping the conversation going

Children in the third year continue to communicate predominantly for social reasons. At the start of this period, conversations with caregivers are often erratic and disjointed. Caregivers assist children to participate for longer in conversations through, for example, responding to what the child has said and at the same time requiring a response from them. Kaye and Charney (1981), cited by Brinton and Fujuki (1989), suggest that the high proportion of these types of caregiver responses, which they term 'turnabouts', was due to the caregiver's role in guiding the interaction, with her main goal being to keep the conversation with her child going.

Children at this stage find it quite hard to enter ongoing nonverbal and verbal interactions with peers, needing to use persistence in order to gain acknowledgement and enter the interaction (Corsaro 1979, cited by Brinton and Fujuki 1989).

Children come to recognize that pauses in conversations function as a signal to take a turn. Ervin-Tripp (1979) cited by Brinton and Fujuki (1989) found that children aged 2 and 3 were less successful than older children in interrupting conversations; apparently, the younger the child, the more likely they were to be ignored. By the time they are 3, children can take a number of turns in a conversation and are increasingly skilled at initiating conversations with others (Examples 3.8, 3.9 and 3.10).

The topic of conversation

As children's linguistic abilities increase during the course of this year, particularly their vocabulary and grammatical skills, so does their ability to maintain the topic of conversation initiated by someone else. They maintain the topic predominantly through imitating what the adult said at the earlier stages, and

Example 3.7 Adapting communication and shifting perspective in role play

Around 29 months, Rowan often initiated a role play game with her mother where they reversed roles, and her mother was required to adopt the role of a baby.

ROWAN: Now you lie down in your cot. *(mother lies on the floor)*
ROWAN: Now you go sleeps. *(mother pretends to sleep)*
MOTHER: Waa! Waa!
ROWAN: What the matter? You want milky? Want your milky?
MOTHER: *(nods)*
ROWAN: I just gonna get your milky.

Ways that Rowan adapted her use of language in the above example include asking her 'baby' if she wants some milk. Outside of a play situation such as this, Rowan would not usually ask adults if they wanted a drink. Also, she uses a derivative form of 'milk' ('milky'), which she only ever used in play, having heard a friend use it in their play scenario. Rowan adopted a solicitous, inquiring tone in her voice, using a higher pitch than normal. This style of intonation was reserved for role play.

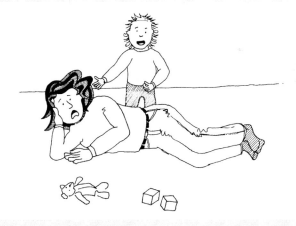

Figure 3.8 Rowan, aged 2½, reverses roles with her mother in pretend play

progress to adding new but related information as they approach their third birthday (Brinton and Fujuki 1989). As in the previous year, adults continue to provide a topical scaffold to conversations with young children. That is, they *expand* on what the child has said by, for example, making a topical connection with past or future events (Wanska and Bedrosian 1986, cited by Brinton and Fujuki 1989) (see Example 3.11).

Example 3.8 Keeping the conversation going

At 26 months old, Rowan had this conversation with her mother, illustrating how Rowan is facilitated to take her turn by the simultaneously acknowledging and requesting nature of her mother's preceding utterance.

ROWAN: Mama take that off. *(hands mother a bag of sweets)*
MOTHER: Shall I open it then?
ROWAN: Yeah, open it. I hold uh bag.
MOTHER: Do you want to hold the bag?
ROWAN: I wanna hold uh bag.

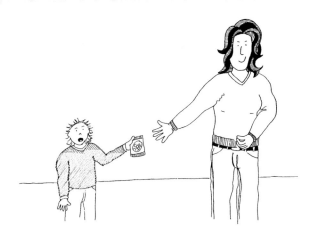

Figure 3.9 Rowan holds a conversation with her mother over a bag of sweets

As they enter their third year, children use their communication skills for a variety of purposes (see Table 2.2, page 64), with the topic of conversation usually focusing on a current activity or on objects or events in the immediate environment. They become gradually more able to talk about topics beyond the here and now, providing a context for learning grammatical forms to express past and future.

Repairing conversations: Responding to requests for clarification

Through the course of this year, children learn to respond with increasing specificity to requests from others (usually adults) for clarification of their messages, demonstrating increasing adaptation to the needs of conversational partners. The most common type of *clarification request* adults tend to use is repetition of part of the child's utterance, with rising intonation (Pan and Snow 1999).

Example 3.9 Successfully initiating a conversation with an adult

At 26 months, Rowan was successful in striking up a conversation with her mother, using persistence, repetition and an increasingly louder voice to gain her mother's attention. At the start of the interaction, Rowan's mother was writing a letter.

ROWAN: Hello.
MOTHER: Hello. *(continues writing)*
ROWAN: I beautiful.
MOTHER: Mmm.
ROWAN: What you doing?
MOTHER: I'm writing. *(head turned towards paper on table)*
ROWAN: Mum, mum, what you doing?
MOTHER: I'm still writing. *(looks up briefly to Rowan, then returns to the letter)*
ROWAN: *(voice getting increasingly loud)* Mum, mum. What you doing? What you doing?
MOTHER: *(picks Rowan up and places her on her knee)* I'm writing a letter, look. Do you want to write something?

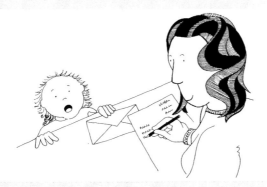

Figure 3.10 Rowan, aged 26 months, strikes up a conversation with her mother

Gallagher (1977), cited by Brinton and Fujuki 1989, found children at 29 months to revise messages by changing or substituting grammatical elements from their original message. An example of this is when a child replaces the pronoun 'it' with the noun phrase 'the chocolate cake' as in the following hypothetical exchange:

CHILD: Can me have it?
MOTHER: Hmm? What do you want?
CHILD: Can me have it?
MOTHER: *(looks puzzled)*
CHILD: Can me have the chocolate cake?

Evidence that children do not merely repeat the message but change it in some way suggests strongly that they appreciate how messages can fail to be conveyed for a number of reasons (Pan and Snow 1999).

Example 3.10 Different ways of initiating conversations

During the course of her third year, Rowan experimented with a number of phrases to initiate a conversation. These included 'Oi!', 'Hey!', 'Mum/Dad' and 'Tell you what'. The most frequently used phrases were the latter two, which were generally highly effective in striking up a conversation.

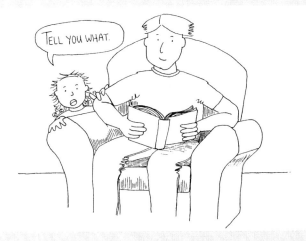

Figure 3.11 Rowan strikes up a conversation with her father

Example 3.11 Expanding on the topic of conversation

ROWAN: Got ears on it.
MOTHER: Who's got ears?
ROWAN: Mummy.
MOTHER: Has Anne got ears?
ROWAN: No. Isn't. Is got hair.

When Rowan was 27 months she had this conversation with her mother, who expanded on the topic of conversation by introducing a new but related element, 'Anne', the name of Rowan's childminder.

Example 3.12 Responding to a request for clarification

At 30 months, Rowan showed her mother a picture she had completed at her playgroup.

ROWAN: It got sticky on it.
MOTHER: *(mishearing)* It's got *sweeties* on it?
ROWAN: No! It got sticky on it.

Rowan responded to her mother's request for clarification by stressing the word sticky using increased loudness and a higher pitched voice.

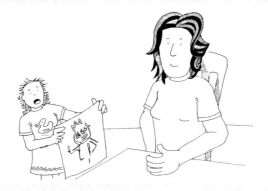

Figure 3.12 Rowan clarifies what she says, aged 2½

Repairing conversations: making requests for clarification

Children also make requests for clarification from conversational partners. Mostly at this age they employ neutral strategies such as 'What?' or 'Hmm?', or repeat part of the speaker's utterance. However, children make these requests far less frequently than do adults, and almost not at all with peers (Pan and Snow 1999).

Requests for clarification form a relatively high proportion of utterances addressed to children at this stage. With the topic of such exchanges being language itself and the goal being to encourage children to reflect on the effectiveness of their messages, Pan and Snow (1999) suggest that caregivers are now responding to children's higher level of language abilities by holding them more accountable for what they say.

Further uses of language in the third year

The considerable advances children make during their third year in areas such as use of grammatical structures, vocabulary, understanding about the world, social understanding, imagination, attention and memory enable them to use their language skills for an ever-widening range of communicative purposes.

Asking questions

Early on in the third year children become increasingly interested in asking questions. Not only do they continue to use rising intonation on short phrases to ask 'Yes/No' questions such as 'Roro's juice?', 'Go park now?', but they use 'What . . .?' and 'Where . . .?' to seek information about objects and locations of objects (Tager-Flusberg 1989). They have not yet mastered how to ask these questions correctly, but they are certainly able to get their messages across. At these early stages of using 'wh . . .' words (what, where, who, when, why) to ask questions, children are thought to be using a question form, 'What's that', for example, as much as a functional device to engage another person in interaction with them

---

Example 3.13 Asking questions with 'What . . .?'

Around 26 months, Rowan and her mother were playing on the floor when the telephone rang.

ROWAN:　What's that?
MOTHER:　It's the telephone. *(answering the telephone)* Hello?
ROWAN:　What's that? What's that on uh phone?
MOTHER:　It's Clair.

It was not until a few weeks later that she sorted out when to use *what* and when to use *who* in questions.

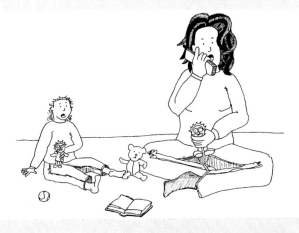

Figure 3.13 Rowan asks, 'What's on the phone?'

(Johnson 1983) as to seek information. They have worked out that asking questions generally secures answers. They are not thought to fully understand the meaning of 'what', in that it refers to an object or thing of some description, and may over use 'What's that' when clearly referring to people, which would require use of 'Who . . .?' Accurate use of 'Who . . .?' to ask questions about people generally occurs a bit later than accurate use of 'What . . .?', and accurate use of the other 'wh' words occurs later still (Tager-Flusberg 1989).

During the second half of this year, children commonly start to ask lots of 'Why..?' questions. As with other 'Wh' questions, they are thought to use 'Why . . .?' as an interaction device to keep conversations going, rather than inquiring after causality, especially in the earlier stages when they do not fully understand the meaning of the word. Answers that adults give to children's 'Why . . .?' questions will help them to arrive at a clearer understanding of the word's meaning.

Expressing feelings, internal states and problems

Words such as 'sad', 'happy', 'cross', 'tired' and 'hungry', which are used to express emotions and internal states, become meaningful over the third year. Children are able to use these words in short phrases to express their own feelings such as 'I sad', 'Me happy', and to begin to talk about how others are feeling.

Example 3.14 Talking about other people's feelings

In her third year, Rowan started to comment on other people's emotions as depicted in television programmes. Soap operas were particularly effective in getting her to say things like:

'Aah . . . poor woman. She sad.'
'She crying. She not happy, mum.'
'Ha ha ha! Silly man. Look uh silly man! She happy, mum.'

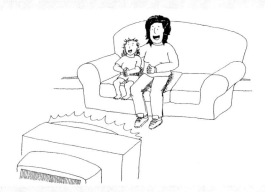

Figure 3.14 Rowan watching television

The emotional development that children experience over the course of the third year can be tumultuous and unpredictable (Leach 1997). Learning how to express feelings using language can only serve to illuminate children's and parents' experiences during this time and make communication more effective.

Example 3.15 Using words to express feelings

Like most other young children, Rowan experienced lots of feelings, including fears, over her third year. Learning words to express how she felt not only assisted her parents in finding out what was wrong and thus how to care for her, but also seemed to help her in understanding her own feelings. Of course, she was not able to use words on every occasion, but when she was able to, this helped her make sense of what she was experiencing. Some examples follow:

'I scared. I scared uh de monsters.'
'I sad. You not my friend. Go 'way.'
'I bit shy uh Grayman. Grayman uh bit shy.' *(Graham was a family friend)*
'You sad, mum?'

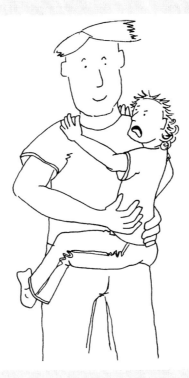

Figure 3.15 Rowan's fears are calmed

Children become better at articulating problems that they are experiencing, especially once they have acquired use of the verbs 'can' and 'cannot'.

Example 3.16 Talking about problems

Rowan became despondent one afternoon as she was playing. She had this conversation with her mother:

ROWAN: Mum. I can't do anything. I can't do it.
MOTHER: What can't you do?
ROWAN: I can't do de puzzle.

Asserting independence

Children at this time are going through the stage often referred to as the 'terrible twos' when they might feel keenly the need to challenge adults' control of them and to assert their own independence (Leach 1997). Phrases such as 'Go 'way', 'Me do it' and 'Lemme!' (for 'let me!') assist children towards finding out about independence.

Talking about the past and future

Children start to use their language to relate what has happened in the past and to express their intentions or wishes for the immediate future. During the third year they start to use the expressions 'wanna', 'gotta', 'gonna' for these purposes, not realizing as yet that they are combinations of two words, for example, 'I wanna go now.' It will be some time yet before they have mastered the necessary grammatical constructions to express past and future with accuracy, but, again, they can be highly successful in getting their messages across.

Early storytelling

Children might start to tell short stories, especially over the second half of this year. Stories will be disjointed and hard to follow initially, and might only be two or three sentences long. Growing vocabulary and grammatical skills help significantly in storytelling, as in picture description, which they get particularly good at towards the end of this year.

Example 3.17 Talking about the past

Rowan and her father returned from a shopping trip and held the following conversation with her mother where she tells about what has recently happened:

ROWAN: I got . . . I got . . . I got . . . shoes! *(points at her new shoes)*
MOTHER: They're lovely. They've got bees on them.
FATHER: Tell mummy what happened in the park.
ROWAN: I fall . . . me cry. Hurt me fingers. *(holds up fingers to be kissed better)*

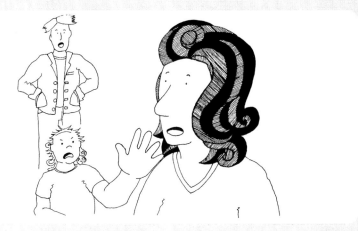

Figure 3.16 Rowan holds her fingers up to be kissed

Developments in expressive language structures

Grammatical development generally occurs once the child's expressive vocabulary has reached on average 300 words (Bates *et al.* 1994, Bates and Goodman 1997), between the ages of 24 and 30 months. Recall from the Introduction (pages 3–4) that grammar refers to the various rules that exist for structuring words and sentences. These include word ending rules for plurals ('cats' vs. 'cat') and *tenses* (*present tense* 'stopping' vs. past tense 'stopped'), and word order rules for expressing different types of sentences (negatives, questions, statements and commands, for example 'You're not painting a picture', 'Are you painting a picture?', 'You're painting a picture' and 'Paint a picture!' respectively). Grammatical development, like other aspects of language development, follows a developmental pattern in English which starts early in the third year. Earliest signs of grammar emerging in children are usually grammatical markers attached to words which alter the word's meaning in some way, as in 'stop', 'stops', 'stopping', 'stopped'. The grammatical

Example 3.18 Talking about the future

Rowan announces her intentions and wishes for the immediate future as follows:

ROWAN: *(approaching a spinning chair)* I wanna go round'n'roun. Now. Now tell you what. *(places herself, doll and toy shopping trolley on chair)* I wanna go round'n'roun.
MOTHER: I'm going to have a bath now. Do you want a bath?
ROWAN: Wanna play this one. *(continues playing with bricks)* *(playing with a doll)* She's wanna go on uh block. *(places doll on a square piece of cloth)*

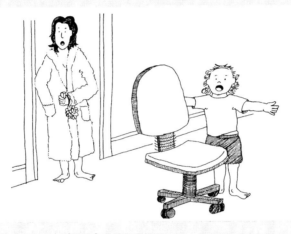

Figure 3.17 Rowan declares her intentions

Example 3.19 Early storytelling

Rowan told the following story to her parents while lying in their bed one morning soon after she woke up:

'There's lion *(extends palm of one hand towards her mother)* . . . and Jeremy Fisher in de other pocket *(extends palm of the other hand towards her mother)* . . . jumping jumping in uh water . . . *(Rowan jumps off the bed)* . . . and lion jumping . . . *(she returns to the bed)* . . . and come back.'

markers are called morphemes – morphemes are the smallest unit of meaning in a language. In order for grammatical development to start, children's expressive vocabulary needs not only to number approximately 300 words, but also to consist of a range of different types of words, such as verbs (action words, for example eating, running, brushing), nouns (names of things, for example apple, dog, house), adjectives (descriptive words, for example big, sticky, cold) and prepositions (positional words, for example in, on).

Three-word phrases emerge between 24 and 30 months

Developments observed in children's conversation skills that occur during this year, in particular the ability to say something that is linked in meaning to the adult's preceding utterance (see pages 96–97) are accompanied by significant advances in children's expressive language skills. The production of three-word phrases that is common during the early part of this year (Tomasello and Brooks 1999) generally occurs once more than half of the child's utterances are two-word phrases. Three-word phrases are usually the result of combinations of two two-word phrases or expansions to a preceding adult utterance (Bloom and Lahey 1978). Each of these is exemplified below.

- *Combinations of two two-word phrases*
  For example, 'Mummy drink' and 'Drink tea' become 'Mummy drink tea'. Before producing this type of three-word phrase, children have usually produced a number of two-word phrases of the type 'Mummy drink', which involves somebody or something that performs an action (for example, mummy), and the action performed (for example, drink). They will also have produced several two-word phrases of the type 'Drink tea' which involves an action (for example, drink) and a thing or person that is acted upon (for example, tea) (Tomasello and Brooks 1999).

- *Expansions to previous sentences spoken by an adult*
  Children expand another person's preceding utterance (Bloom and Lahey 1978), as in the following examples:

  ADULT: Push the car.
  CHILD: Push big car.

  ADULT: This is Daddy's biscuit
  CHILD: No daddy biscuit.

As children first start using three-word phrases they may continue to use a large number of single words and two-word phrases, in addition to gestures. Most of their utterances will continue to be telegraphic for this period, with word order becoming increasingly more accurate and in line with that of adult sentences.

Developments in grammar between 24 and 30 months

Children's phrases start to become more grammatically correct through the gradual use of words such as 'in', 'on', 'he' and 'me' in addition to word endings that alter the word's meaning as in 'Mummy's hat'; 'two cars'; and 'crying'. Table 3.1 outlines the most common developments in grammar that occur during this stage. These developments assist children greatly in specifying more precisely what they intend to say. As in all other areas of language development, there is considerable variability among children regarding ages at which they acquire grammatical structures. Table 3.1 should be used as a general guide for those aspects of grammar that are more likely to be acquired early on.

Developments in grammar between 30 and 36 months

As children approach their third birthdays, their expressive language becomes far less telegraphic, with much more consistent use of grammatical structures acquired earlier in the year. It will still take a considerable time before children make no grammatical errors, however. There continue to be several errors, especially on verb forms such as past tense construction (for example 'we goed to the park'), the auxiliary verbs 'can' and 'will' and various forms of the verb 'to be' (am, are, is). Children's sentences get longer, especially once they start to use linking words like 'and' and 'because'. There may be up to three or four separate pieces of information, or key words in single sentences. Table 3.2 summarizes the grammatical structures commonly used over this stage; once again, the table should act as a general guide only, bearing in mind the wide variability that exists among children regarding rate of language acquisition.

What do children's errors tell us about how they learn language?

Errors that children make as they go through the process of acquiring language provide lots of evidence that they are active learners, testing out hypotheses and constantly re-evaluating their efforts in response to feedback they receive (Tager-Flusberg 1989). The fact that so many of their utterances contain errors is proof enough that they do not learn language through imitation of what adults say, but through testing out grammatical rules and meanings of words until they arrive at accurate use. Some child language researchers (Roeper 1982, in Tager-Flusberg 1989) support the notion that children have an innate predisposition to learn the grammar of their ambient language – the errors they make in applying grammatical rules is testament to there being an underlying facility for analyzing, and thus learning the form, or structure of a language.

Many 3-year-old children are able to analyze different types of phrase structures within sentences (Roeper 1982). Roeper discusses how 3-year-olds respond differentially to the sentences:

Table 3.1 Common features of grammatical development between 24 and 30 months

Grammatical structure	Examples from Rowan's speech during her third year
Pronouns I, me, it, him	I sad. I wanna go now. Oh, it beautiful. It uh man.
Prepositions In, on	Mustn't stand on it. I putting rabbit in there. I put in my pocket.
-ing *verb* ending	That uh man – look, she standing. Daddy sleeping.
Future aspect Wanna, gonna, gotta	I wanna play this one. She's gonna get cold.
Plural Regular -s ending	Look mum, doggies! I got toys.
Negative No, not	I not happy. I not comb my hair. There no pig here.
Questions What, where	What that? Where daddy go?

Sources: Tager-Flusberg (1989) and Brown (1973).

Table 3.2 Common features of grammatical development between 30 and 36 months

Grammatical structure	Examples from Rowan's speech during her third year
Pronouns I, he, she, you, they, we	I can see it. You make uh bubbles. He's want a chair. I put them up there. She's not sleepy.
Verbs Can, will, be	I can watch. I can see it. This is my book. She *is* sleepy; There *is*.
Verb endings Regular past	I pushed it. Stopped now. Cat jumped off.
Plural Regular -s ending more consistent	Two foots. She's got boots on.
Negatives Can't, don't, not, no used mid-sentence	I don't like it. Daddy didn't got yellow one. Daddy's not got yellow one. I not want crisps.
Questions Who, why	Who that at uh door? Why you working, dad?
Articles The, a	I going in a front room . . . you going in a front room? Get the brush then, use the brush. Look, it's a comb, it's beautiful hair, it's a nice hair.
Conjunctions And, because	Tidy up now 'cos it bathtime. I go playgroup and . . . and . . . and I did painting.

Sources: Tager-Flusberg (1989) and Brown (1973).

1   I hit the boy with my hand.
2   I hit the boy with a hat.

They were able to give appropriate answers to the question, 'Who did you hit?' for each sentence. These are 'The boy' (and not 'the boy with my hand') and 'The boy with a hat' respectively. This provides evidence that they have analyzed the relevant types of phrases accurately. The difference in the types of phrases for each of the sentences is that sentence 1 'with my hand' is not part of the same noun phrase as 'the boy', while in sentence 2 'with a hat' can be.

Overgeneralization

Children frequently *overgeneralize* grammatical rules, such as:

- applying plural '-s' ending to words like 'foot' and 'mouse' as in Rowan's utterance 'Two foots'
- over-use of a particular pronoun, as in Rowan's use of 'she' for both 'he' and 'she' – 'Look uh silly man! She happy.'
- over-use of the regular past tense ending '-ed' as in, 'We just buyed them.'

Semantic errors

Children continue to make errors related to word meanings well into their school years. It is not uncommon for children during their third year to invent new ways for using common words, such as in the following examples:

- 'Mum, I gonna fall it' (Rowan aged 28 months about to drop a toy)
- 'Don't giggle me', 'Don't uncomfortable the cat' (Bowerman 1982, cited by Roeper 1982).

These types of errors suggest that children need to continue learning about the limitations of word meanings, and how words can be combined with each other, in order to express meanings accurately.

Speech development

Once again, it is important to stress the wide variability that exists among children regarding ages at which aspects of speech development occur, in addition to variability regarding the order in which sounds are acquired. The information contained in the following sections should be used as a general guide only.

Main changes that occur in speech

The main changes affecting children's speech over the third year are that children use a wider range of speech sounds and fewer simplification patterns than previously.

Recall from Chapter 2 (pages 75–76) that children in the early stages of speech development omit parts of words or some sounds, and they use easier sounds in place of more difficult ones. In the third year there is also less variability in how words sound, relative to adult pronunciations (Stackhouse and Wells 1997).

Most children this age have not yet developed the ability to analyse the separate components of words such as sounds and syllables; their knowledge about these aspects of words depends on how familiar the word is. Children are better at listening out for the difference in how pairs of words sound when the words are familiar ('back' and 'bag') than when they are less familiar ('frock' and 'frog') (Stackhouse and Wells 1997). As children's vocabularies develop, so does the ability to identify similarities and differences in how different words sound. An example of this is awareness about *rhyme* (for example an awareness that the two words 'mouse' and 'house' have the same ending). The development of this and related skills is gradual, however, and continues over the next few years. Refer to the section '*Phonological awareness*' in Chapter 4 (page 146) for more discussion on the nature and development of these skills.

Simplification patterns in the third year

Most simplification patterns that children use at the start of this year are the same ones that children use towards the end of the second year. They affect the word as a whole, rather than selected sounds within the word (Grunwell 1987, Stackhouse and Wells 1997). Examples of these two types of simplification patterns are given in the following paragraphs, and in Table 3.3. Simplification patterns that affect selected sounds, or groups of sounds, become more common as children develop over this year, and many of these remain until the ages of 6 or 7. Of course, children differ enormously in their use of simplification patterns. Simultaneous use of several simplification patterns, especially those which affect the word as a whole, results in speech that is more difficult to understand.

Table 3.3 Examples of simplification processes commonly applied during the third year

Target word	Child's pronunciation	Simplification process
tomato	mato	weak syllable deletion
bed	be	final consonant deletion
tickle	kickle	consonant harmony
stop	top	's' blend reduction (st → t)
crisps	kip	reduction of blends other than 's' (here, cr → k)
top, pip, cook	dop, bip, gook	context sensitive voicing
fan, sun	pan, tun	stopping
key, gate	tea, date	fronting
run, yellow	wun, lellow	gliding

The most common simplification patterns in the third year are discussed in the following paragraphs. Some children might use simplification patterns that are not covered in this book, and some children develop their own idiosyncratic patterns. Table 3.3 provides examples of simplification patterns commonly used during the third year.

Simplification patterns affecting the word as a whole

This type of pattern affects the overall 'shape' of the word, commonly by omitting part of the word, with the result that the word is shorter and contains fewer syllables and sounds than the adult version.

Patterns that generally fade out towards the end of the third year:

- 'final consonant deletion', for example dog → do; bed → be
- 'consonant harmony' – initial syllables are repeated, for example dolly → dodo, or a single consonant replaces two or more consonants, for example tiger → giger
- 'context sensitive voicing' – all consonants at the beginnings of words are pronounced with activation of the vocal folds to produce voice, for example table → dable; pear → bear.

Patterns that are common in children this and the following year:

- 'weak syllable deletion' – unstressed syllable is omitted, for example 'mato' for 'tomato'
- 'reduction of 's' blends', for example spoon → boon.

Pattern that occurs well into the fourth year, and sometimes later:

- 'reduction of blends other than 's'', for example grandma → ganma; present → pesent.

Simplification patterns affecting individual sounds or groups of sounds

- '*Stopping*' is the name given to the process where sounds made by air being forced through a narrow gap in the mouth area (fricatives – f, v, th, s, z, sh) are replaced by 'stops'. Stops are sounds made where air is built up in the mouth and suddenly released explosively (for example p, b, d, t, k, g). All fricatives may be 'stopped' during this year; it is usual for 'f' and 's' to be pronounced accurately towards the end of the third year, however.
- '*Fronting*' is the name given to the process where sounds that are normally made with the back of the tongue touching the palate (k, g, ng) are replaced by sounds made with the tongue tip touching the hard ridge of bone behind the top front teeth (t, d).

• '*Gliding*' is a very common process used by most children of this age. Gliding may persevere through to late childhood (and may not even resolve in adulthood), and involves the sounds 'l' and 'r' being pronounced as 'y' and 'w' respectively.

Range of sounds commonly produced over the third year

Generally, by the age of 3, children have increased their inventories of speech sounds to include the following: m, p, b, w, n, t, d, k, g, ng, h, f, s, y and possibly l. This advance means that their speech is far easier to understand. This is important, as by now most children have a lot to say, have developed large vocabularies and are using longer utterances. It is more difficult to understand what someone with immature or unusual pronunciation is saying if they are using long sentences and lots of different words.

Developmental dysfluency in the third year

Some children experience disruptions to their speech fluency over the third year, often related to simultaneous advances made in their language development. Further discussion on developmental dysfluency can be found on page 144.

Summary of Chapter 3

Attention control

1   Children's control over their own focus of attention becomes gradually more flexible, but remains mostly single-channelled.

Links between play and language

2   Children start to use their imagination in play; objects used in symbolic play might bear little perceptual similarity to those they represent.
3   Towards the end of the third year, children become engaged in play with peers.

Conceptual, semantic and vocabulary development

4   The size of children's vocabularies is greatly affected by the amount of words they hear.
5   Children start to understand the groupings that exist among words, and develop their understanding of words relating to basic concepts.

Understanding words and sentences

6 Children rely less on nonlinguistic information to comprehend spoken language; they still make use of strategies involving 'doing what you normally do', however.

7 Children's receptive vocabularies include names of all common objects, actions, adjectives and prepositions.

8 Children develop the ability to process and follow instructions containing up to three key words.

9 Children understand and use question forms 'what', 'where', 'who', and 'why'.

Communication and expressive skills in the third year

10 Conversation skills develop so that children are able to use and respond effectively to a number of conversational strategies:

- they are able to initiate conversations, especially with adults
- they can increasingly adjust what they say in response to different listeners' needs, which is closely linked to a developing ability to see things from a point of view other than their own
- they become more adept at maintaining a topic of conversation
- they start to talk about a wider range of subjects, including past and possibly future events.

11 Children come to use language for an increasing range of purposes including asking questions, expressing feelings and early storytelling.

12 Children's utterances contain three-word phrases and, once expressive vocabulary has reached 300 words, morphemes appear.

13 Towards the end of the third year sentence length further increases by use of 'and' and 'because'; past tense, plurals, negatives and questions are expressed through use of relevant grammatical structures.

14 Children make developmental errors when selecting words and constructing sentences.

Speech development

15 Children use simplification patterns when pronouncing words; these increasingly affect groups of sounds rather than the word as a whole towards the end of the year. Speech is clear, though immature, by the age of 3.

Key skills 3.1 Communication skills usually achieved by 2½-year-old children

- Relies increasingly on words to express self, but still uses gesture and other nonverbal behaviours
- Takes two or three turns in conversations with listener
- Enacts familiar activities in play (for example with dolls)
- Verbal commentary accompanies play
- Watches peers at play and occasionally joins in
- Focus of attention often rigid on absorbing activity; gradually increasing flexibility in attention control
- Uses strategy of doing what is usually done when responding to instructions (for example 'Put the knife on the plate')
- Recognizes names and pictures of most common objects
- Identifies objects by function (for example 'Which one is for eating?')
- Understands 'What?' and 'Where?'
- Understands sentences with three key words (for example 'Get a *biscuit* and your *big beaker*')
- Average size of expressive vocabulary is 500 words
- Starting to use three-word phrases (for example 'Eat mummy cake')
- Asks lots of questions with 'What?' and 'Where?'
- Starts talking about events in the past and, occasionally, the future
- Starts to use grammatical structures:

  - plural -s (doggies, toys)
  - pronouns (I, me, it)
  - negative (I not happy, no juice)

- Single words and short phrases should be clear, though immature

Before using this table, see page xxi.

Key skills 3.2 Communication skills usually achieved by 3-year-old children

- Uses language as the main means of communicating
- Takes a number of turns in conversation
- Initiates conversations and is increasingly able to maintain topic of conversation
- Imagination evident in play; attributes imaginary entities with properties (for example produces imaginary cat from pocket for adult to stroke, says the cat is hungry)
- Enacts less familiar events in play (for example visit to dentist, zoo)
- Becomes involved in sustained make-believe play with peers
- Able to shift focus of attention from activity she is engaged in to verbal direction and back to activity, but needs adult support to do so
- Uses strategy of offering explanation for questions not understood
- Understands all common action words, object names, most common adjectives
- Understands 'Who?', 'Whose?', 'Why?' and occasionally 'How many?'
- Follows instructions containing three, sometimes four, key words (for example 'Find the *big beaker* and put it in *Johnny's bag*')
- Understands many words referring to basic concepts (for example in, on, under, big, small, long, short)
- Expressive vocabulary consists on average of 700 words
- Asks questions using 'Why?'
- Talks increasingly about the past and future; tells short, often disjointed, stories
- Uses grammatical structures:

  - pronouns (*I, he, she, you, they, we*)
  - verbs (*can, will, is, are*)
  - verb endings (*pushed, stopped*)
  - negatives mid sentence (*I not like it*)
  - articles (*a, the*)
  - conjunctions (*and, because*)

- Speech is mostly understandable, with some continuing immaturities

Before using this table, see page xxi.

Warning signs 3.1 Possible warning signs for 2½-year-old children

- **Withdrawn or quiet on a consistent basis**
- **Poor socially and does not appear to want to play with adult**
- **Little pretend or imaginative play**
- **Never concentrates on anything for more than a few seconds**
- **Difficulty identifying names of common objects without gesture**
- **Difficulty following simple instructions (for example 'Come here' without gesture)**
- **Unable to follow two key words in sentences (for example 'Put teddy on the chair')**
- **Only uses single words in utterances**
- **Continuing to rely on pointing and other gesture to get what she wants**
- **Number of words she uses is not growing**
- **Continuing to babble, using sentence-like melody**
- **Stammering**
- **Speech is very difficult to understand to unfamiliar adults**
- **Parents express concerns, are worried or anxious**

⚠ See below.

Warning signs 3.2 Possible warning signs for 3-year-old children

- **Not showing interest in playing with peers**
- **Poor social skills**
- **Very limited awareness of what others know and what needs to be explained when talking to others**
- **Not very good at or interested in holding conversations**
- **Never concentrates on anything for more than a few seconds**
- **Little pretend or imaginative play**
- **Often shows signs of not understanding what has been said**
- **Shows no interest in stories**
- **Often says things that are irrelevant or inappropriate to the situation; repeats same learned phrase or sentence out of context**
- **Still only using single words or phrases consisting of two words**
- **Does not ask questions**
- **Stammering**
- **Speech is very difficult to understand, sometimes even for familiar adults**
- **Parents express concerns, are worried or anxious**

⚠ Before using this table, see page xxii.

The fourth and fifth years

4

O Key areas of language development; links with developments in attention, play, socialization and cognition.

O The role of conversation as a context for language development, and uses of language.

O Links between spoken and written language.

O Impact of television and video viewing on communication, attention and play development.

O Summary of key points; tables of communication skills usually achieved in the fourth and fifth years; tables of possible warning signs to help identify children with communication difficulties.

Attention control

Attention control in the fourth year

Gradually over the course of the fourth year, children begin to control their own focus of attention. They become able to shift attention from what they are currently engaged in to what a speaker is saying without needing an adult to cue them in by saying their name, for example. It still takes a bit of time before the child is able successfully to achieve a shift of focus, especially if she is engaged in a particularly absorbing activity. Attention remains single-channelled in that the child is not able to attend to what a speaker is saying if it does not relate to what she is currently doing. Children at this stage still need adequate preparation for changes in activity and enough time to make a shift in focus of attention. The big step is that she is able to shift her attention spontaneously and under her own control, moving gradually towards the stage where she only needs to look at the speaker if the speaker's language becomes hard to understand (Cooper *et al.* 1978).

Attention control in the fifth year

Over the course of this year, there is gradual integration of the auditory and visual channels until the child is capable of fully integrated attention. She is then able to listen and respond appropriately to instructions without looking up or stopping what she is doing. Achievement of integrated attention occurs in small steps at first, with the concentration span increasing as the child matures (Cooper *et al.* 1978). When children have achieved this level of attention control they are ready for learning in a classroom, where instructions are often given by a teacher to a group of children currently engaged in an activity or task of some description. Attending in a classroom presents challenges for children who have not developed the necessary attention control, as there are many distractions available in the form of other children, environmental noises and interesting things to look at out of the window or on the walls.

Links between play and language

The major change that occurs in play development over the fourth and fifth years is that it becomes an increasingly social activity with an ever-greater reliance on effective interaction and language skills. The functions of play over these years build on those of the previous year to include:

- the further development of abstract thought
- the facilitation of peer relationships and friendships
- the enactment of a child's understanding of the world, in particular her understanding of social relationships
- supporting later literacy development and school achievement through the development of *narrative* skills, i.e. the *decontextualized* ordering and categorizing of real or imagined events.

(Garvey 1977, Hetherington and Parke 1986)

Once again, pretend and role play, which are considered to have close links to language development, will be considered here.

The components of pretend play in the preschool years

Roles and identities

Half-way through the fourth year, children become more adept at adopting roles other than 'I' (Hetherington and Parke 1986). This enables them to explore the more familiar family roles (baby, sibling, mother, father, husband, wife) and less familiar 'functional' roles (cook, driver, teacher, fireman, policeman, doctor). Some 3-year-olds are able to remain in role with a playmate for up to 15 minutes at a time, only occasionally slipping out of role (Garvey 1977). Role play that involves differentiated roles such as cook and diner, driver and passenger, mummy and baby, provides opportunities for encouraging social play among groups of children.

Plans for actions and storylines

Garvey (1977) identified a limited number of common themes preschool children enact in pretend play – treating and healing, averting threat, cooking, eating, fixing, telephoning, packing and going on trips. The children she observed were seen to construct their play scenarios around these commonly recurring themes. Events and storylines in pretend play are not thought to be copied from real events as such. Garvey discusses Vygotsky's theory that those features of the world which are currently most salient for children at a given time are more likely to be highlighted and represented in some way through pretend play enactments. Invented actions that children cannot have possibly experienced but which they have been able to infer from their knowledge about the world are commonly observed in pretend play. Examples include role playing adults and animals, and engaging in fantasy play. The limited range of themes in pretend play is thought to help a child's ability to recognize storylines. This facilitates shared involvement and permits planning and enactment of storylines which can be elaborated upon in line with players' communicative and imaginative abilities (Garvey 1977).

Objects and settings

As most children approach their third birthdays, their pretend play remains partly dependent on the objects that are available in the immediate environment. Telephones and cookers will encourage play scenarios around talking on the telephone and cooking. However, as children become better at operating with roles and plans, their pretend play becomes less dependent on the properties of objects. Well-formed pretend play is not considered to take place before the age of 3 (Garvey 1977). During the fourth and fifth years, pretend play is mostly based around ideas that children communicate, whereas prior to this stage it was mostly based around objects in the immediate physical environment. Pretend play that involves making associations between things, people, actions and words, and manipulating and recombining these, supports not only the development of social skills, but also of abstract thought during the fourth and fifth years.

The role of communication skills in play

Communication skills are fundamental to the development of play during this period. As pretend play moves increasingly towards becoming a social activity that is based on ideas, the need for social interaction skills and the ability to understand and communicate ideas becomes greater.

Example 4.1 Use of imagination in play

A few months before her fourth birthday, Rowan was playing a game with her mother that developed out of her ideas and her imagination. Use of props (for example the horns) is limited but highly flexible.

MOTHER: The ghost isn't going to come down here.
ROWAN: It will.
MOTHER: How do you know?
ROWAN: It will . . . it's coming through the door.
MOTHER: What's that noise?
ROWAN: It's . . . I think it's a ghost.
MOTHER: I'm not sure.
ROWAN: It is . . . let's not play that game again . . . it's too scared.
MOTHER: How about if . . .
ROWAN: If the ghost turns into a frog! Frog!
MOTHER: Shall we go and have a look, see if it's turned into a magic frog?
ROWAN: No! We need a magic wand!
MOTHER: Oh look! There's something. *(points to a balloon on a stick)*
ROWAN: It hasn't got any magic! It's got air!
MOTHER: Let's go find a magic wand then.
ROWAN: *(looking in a box)* Here's my horns! *(she had needed these when being a butterfly the previous day)*
MOTHER: That's for when you're a butterfly – let's go and find that frog.
ROWAN: Got to turn it into a frog. Can I be a butter . . . a magic butterfly. Now this is magic. *(puts horns on her head)*
MOTHER: OK, you be the magic butterfly.
ROWAN: Magic, magic . . . oh big frog!
MOTHER: It's turned into a big frog! Oh look, it's hopping down the stairs.
ROWAN: *(squealing and laughing)* Look! It's poking through the stairs! *(uses a deep, 'frog' voice)* Allo! Allo! Ribbet! Ribbet!
MOTHER: Are you a friendly frog?
ROWAN: Yes. I think it's our pet.

Links between play, social interaction and friendship formation

Hetherington and Parke (1986) and Garvey (1977) draw links between the development of positive social interaction skills, skilled enactment of pretend play and popularity amongst peers. Positive interaction skills cited by Garvey (1977: 158) are 'being attentive to the purpose at hand and responsive to others, contributing positively to the ongoing action, and communicating clearly and relevantly'. Children who display these skills are more successful at entering ongoing play between two or more children, especially unfamiliar peers (Garvey 1977). The roles of positive interaction and clear communication skills become crucial in successful make-believe play between two or more children. Joining in play with others is central to children's social relationships, and therefore their social development. Joining in the play of other children, which is expected to occur after the age of 3, is largely dependent on a child's ability to interact with others and to use communication skills effectively.

Garvey discusses Gottman's studies (Garvey 1977) that explore the process of friendship formation in young children. During early childhood, friendships develop largely through involvement in mutually enjoyable play. The more the children are in tune with or interpersonally coordinated with the other, the more enjoyable and entertaining the play. Garvey agrees with Gottman's claim (Garvey 1977: 156) that the highest level of coordinated play is fantasy play, which cannot be achieved without 'continuous interpersonal monitoring, clear and appropriate communication, whole-hearted involvement, and a willingness to compromise'. Play among friends, including fantasy play which by its very nature is vulnerable to a high number of disputes and disagreements, involves a higher number of coordinated phrases involving 'let's' and 'we', and a higher proportion of agreements to disagreements in their language.

The range of communicative functions expressed through play

In order for pretend play to be coordinated among a number of children, there needs to be explicit talk about plans, roles, objects and settings involved in the play. Children need not only to be able to slip between familiar roles, but also to announce that they are doing so. Players need to be kept abreast of developments in the plan through clear direction of scenes. The greater a child's range of communicative functions, the greater is the likelihood that the play episode will be coordinated, understood, and therefore enjoyed among players. Children need to be able to make a range of statements ('I'm the mummy and you're the baby'; 'This is the car'; 'You're on the train and I'm in the buggy'), give and take directions ('Now you give me the dummy'; 'Put the monster in the mud'; 'It's time for you to run away') ask questions, make suggestions and give descriptions.

The role of pragmatics in pretend play

The enactment of pretend play calls for the creative use of a range of pragmatic skills. Adopting different identities requires children to act and speak in ways that are consistent with particular roles. Pretending to be 'the teacher' involves acting and speaking as a teacher, reacting to children as a teacher might and expressing appropriate ideas and attitudes. Garvey notes that certain features of enactment are highly stereotyped, while others are highly realistic. For example, when enacting mothers speaking to babies, children are observed to use characteristics of speech that adults often use when speaking to young children. Briefly, these include using shorter and simplified sentences, a higher pitch of voice, increased use of endearments, repetitions, and referring to oneself in the third person – 'You hungry, baby? Are you? Hungry girl? You're a hungry girl. Mummy give you milky now.'

Pretend play, narrative and school achievement

The importance of narrative to school achievement

Narrative is the telling of real or fictional past events (which are notable for being unusual or unexpected), that are related in time through a series of causes and effects, that pose a problem or difficulty that needs overcoming, that involve one or more characters, and that end with a resolution of the problem and a final evaluation. Development of narrative skills involves understanding and generating language that is decontextualized, or at a *discourse* level (in spoken language) and *text* level (in written language). Understanding of narrative does not therefore rely on the listener's or reader's immediate environment. This type of language use becomes increasingly important as children progress through school and need to learn to understand and produce many different kinds of texts, as well as to engage in discourse in a variety of situations for a variety of purposes (Garvey 1977).

Refer to relevant sections further on in this chapter (pages 135–139 and 145), which outline the development of narrative skills between the ages of 3 and 5, and the significance of narrative skills in linking spoken and written language.

Links between pretend play and narrative

Pretend play and narrative have much in common. Both take place within a 'frame' that may be explicitly announced or introduced, and appropriate information is then given about the setting and characters, or roles. A sequence of ordered events is then presented, frequently involving a problem of some sort, such as being eaten by lions or the baby falling out of her buggy. A resolution to the problem is then necessary, ending with evaluative judgements on the outcome. The pragmatic and linguistic skills that are necessary for successful cooperative pretend play are also necessary for successful understanding and production of narrative (Garvey 1977). In both cases, speakers need to make appropriate assumptions about what the listeners or players know about the chosen subject matter, or topic, and furnish additional information, for example on the setting, as appropriate. Equally, they need to make appropriate assumptions about what listeners or players might expect to happen in a given situation, and provide an appropriate amount of information in order that communication is effective in the play scenario or narrative.

There are also similarities between the language structures used in the pretend play of 4- and 5-year-olds and those that are commonly found in narratives. Garvey discusses Pellegrini's study (Garvey 1977), which discovered 4- and 5-year-old children's increased use of these language structures in pretend play – use of pronouns to refer to previously introduced objects or characters (for example he, she, it); use of temporal and causal *conjunctions* (for example next, then, finally, because, so); use of elaborated noun phrases (for example the woman with the enormous bag; the big, fat silver snake); use of *future* and past tense verbs (for example, I'm gonna eat you up; you didn't catch me – you caught the lion).

The impact of the media culture on play and language development

The impact of television and videos on play development

Levin's work (1998) forces careful consideration of how the media culture impacts on children's development. She draws close links between the violence, stereotyping and commercialism that characterize so many children's television programmes and lower levels of imagination, creativity and problem-solving in many children's play.

Carlsson-Paige and Levin (1990) have reported changes in the nature of children's play that they also relate directly to violent play themes in the media. These changes include greater fascination with war play and with merchandise from programmes which encourage this type of play, higher levels of aggressive behaviour evident in imitative play based on programmes with violent themes, and reduced creativity and imagination in play.

In the face of negative criticism of much of children's television, it is also important to point out how age-appropriate programmes and videos with non-violent themes can positively influence children's pretend play. They provide a storyline that can be followed (usually quite rigidly by younger children) or extended in an imaginative way (especially by older children and with sensitive adult input). They provide opportunities to try out new words, rhymes and songs, albeit in a context-bound way initially. They enable children to take on different roles and to use narrative and negotiation skills with each other as the play is established and progresses. Different children might have different interpretations of characters and the plot. In these ways, enactment with peers and/or adults of favourite programmes and video stories paves children's way for later involvement in literature and drama.

The impact of television and videos on language, communication and attention development

There are potentially positive and negative aspects to young children watching television programmes and videos. Healy (1998) warns against too much television viewing, stating that repeated exposure to any stimulus can forcibly impact mental and emotional development through influencing the course of brain development or by depriving it of other types of experiences. She states:

While appropriate stimuli – close interaction with loving caregivers; an enriched, interactive, human language environment; engrossing hands-on play opportunities; and age-appropriate academic stimulation – enhance the brain's development, environments that encourage intellectual passivity and maladaptive behaviour (e.g. impulsivity, violence), or deprive the brain of important chances to participate actively in social relationships, creative play, reflection and complex problem-solving may have deleterious and irrevocable consequences.

(Healy 1998)

Healy draws a link between high levels of television viewing and low academic achievement, particularly in reading scores. She speculates that the powerful visual nature of the television stimulus negatively impinges on the development of areas of the brain responsible for language development. She also speculates on television's negative impact on development of attention and listening skills, especially for language, and comments on how the 'two-minute mind' has low tolerance for subject matter requiring depth of processing. Healy suggests that the nature of many features of children's television programmes (for example flashes of colour, quick movement in the peripheral visual field and sudden loud noises) predisposes some children to developing attention problems. In her experience as a paediatrician, some children diagnosed with attention deficit disorder markedly improved once television viewing was reduced.

However, it is impracticable to ban television for children, and many programmes provide important cultural references that serve as topics of conversation and thus a focus of interaction and play, especially for older children. The views of speech and language therapists Bell (1998), Watters (1998), Dunseath (1998) and Taylor (1998) on children's television are summarized below:

- Programmes should be viewed with a parent who can follow up viewing with their child by playing games, singing songs and jointly doing related activities as a basis for conversation (Dunseath 1998).
- Some programmes model appropriate early interaction and language skills such as taking turns, waiting for each other, giving each other time to talk, taking time to listen and lots of repetitious, functional language (Bell 1998).
- Some programmes promote early vocabulary learning and extend knowledge about words, basic concepts, rhyme and music, while being enjoyable at the same time (Bell 1998). Parents are encouraged to identify programmes which provide a good mix of stories, songs, role play and creative activities, and watch these with their children (Dunseath 1998).
- Selected videos can encourage early communication skills and later language development through the use of repetition, imitation and imaginative play (Watters 1998). It is essential that parents encourage their children to interact socially and do not rely on television and video to provide company for them.
- Many videos relate to books, which can be positive in encouraging reading and book sharing. Like favourite story books, some children's videos reveal more and more of themselves with repeated viewing.

- Bell (1998), Watters (1998), Dunseath (1998) and Taylor (1998) are in agreement that it is more realistic and productive to encourage parents to think about how television and videos might be used most effectively for communication and language development, rather than ordering no television for children.

Semantic and vocabulary development

By the age of 4, children have mastered understanding and use of all basic grammatical structures, yet will continue to expand their vocabularies throughout their lives. As with adults, the number of words that children understand far exceeds the number they use.

At approximately 5 years of age, the number of words that children are able to use (their expressive vocabulary) reaches on average 5,000 (Paul and Miller 1995). Children's understanding of less frequently heard words increases significantly as they reach the age of 5. Children may appear to understand some words in one context but not in another (French and Nelson 1985, cited by Myers Pease *et al.* 1989). The 3- and 4-year-olds they studied were able to use the words 'before' and 'after' correctly when talking about familiar events in their own lives, but children of the same age had difficulties carrying out instructions involving the same words in a testing situation. Children's knowledge of what usually happens in a given situation aided or hampered their comprehension of sentences like 'When a girl feeds a baby before putting it to bed' and 'When a girl puts a baby to bed before picking up a pencil' (Myers Pease *et al.* 1989). As at previous stages, factors including the language that children hear around them play an important role in development of children's vocabularies.

With age and increasing cognitive maturity, children's ability to relate words meaningfully to other words develops. Building on their developing knowledge of the groupings that exist among words (for example, 'cows', 'dogs', 'sheep', 'pigs' all belong to the category of 'animals'), children's understanding of word meanings becomes increasingly differentiated and closer to the adult's meaning. This development is accompanied by children being able to provide increasingly specific definitions of words (Myers Pease *et al.* 1989, Johnson 2000). Prior to the age of 4½, children do not provide any defining features of words when asked questions like 'What's a key?' or 'What's a cousin?' They might respond instead by providing some information from their personal experience of keys and cousins – 'I have a cousin Daniel', or 'Mummy's got keys' (after Haviland and Clark 1974, in Myers Pease *et al.* 1989). At around 4½, many children can be expected to provide definitions of words by their function. Haviland and Clark asked a boy of 5 years 10 months 'What's a father?', who responded with, 'A father is somebody who goes to work every day except Saturday and Sunday and earns money.' Of course, children's different experiences will continue to influence their understanding of word meanings to some extent.

Clark's semantic feature hypothesis (in Myers Pease *et al.* 1989) contributes towards explaining the gradual build up in word meaning that children develop over the years. This hypothesis suggests that the adult's understanding of word meanings is composed of sets of features that together uniquely define words. Words may share some features, but no two words will have the exact set. The word 'lettuce' shares many features with other words such as 'cabbage' and 'cauliflower' but is alone in its unique set, as shown in Figure 4.1.

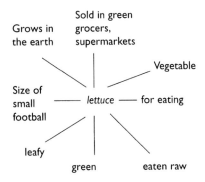

Figure 4.1 Semantic features of 'lettuce'

As children's vocabularies develop, so the number of semantic features defining each word increases, more closely matching the adult meaning, with the result that overextension of word use gradually reduces (Myers Pease *et al.* 1989). Where a younger child might have used the word 'lettuce' to refer to lettuces, cabbages and cauliflowers, the same child will most likely have learned to apply the correct labels by the age of 5, providing they have had experience of these items.

After the age of 5, children's understanding of word meanings and their ability to use words appropriately in different contexts continue to develop as their vocabularies grow. As they mature, children come to link and define words using relational concepts (opposites, similes, explanations), providing abstract definitions over functional definitions (Myers Pease *et al.* 1989).

Understanding words and sentences

Between the ages of 3 and 5, children's understanding of language becomes quite advanced and they appear to understand almost everything they hear. There is a sharp increase (75 per cent) in the proportion of conversational responses 3½-year-olds make that are topically linked to what the speaker has just said (Bloom, Rocissano and Hood 1976, in Paul 1995). This suggests that by this age children are better at analyzing and understanding the language that is spoken to them.

Use of comprehension strategies

Children's ability to process linguistic input more accurately is evidenced by a reduced use of the comprehension strategies typical of younger children when asked to carry out instructions, and when responding to questions in conversations. The 'probable event' and 'supplying missing information' strategies discussed in Chapter 3 continue to be used by children of this age group. Marinac and Ozanne (1999) have specified a developmental hierarchy for the use of comprehension strategies by children aged between 3 and 4½. 'Supplying missing information' (or 'random answering') was discovered to be the most commonly used strategy by children aged between 3 and 3½. For example, while children are still working out the relative meanings of the more advanced '*Wh-*' *question words* (why, how and when) they may continue to respond to 'Wh-' questions by answering as if another question had been asked (James 1990, in Paul 1995). So a child might respond to the question, 'How did you get to school?' by saying, 'With mummy'.

The 'probable event' strategy was most commonly used by all children aged between 3 and 4½, and involves the child making a response which is related in meaning to what the speaker has said, and leads to the most usual or typical action. If a child within this age group interpreted an improbable sentence such as 'The baby feeds the mummy' as 'The mummy feeds the baby', they would be following the normal pattern of development, despite being incorrect in their literal understanding of the language (Paul 1995).

The third comprehension strategy analysed by Marinac and Ozanne (1999), that of 'semantic probability', was found to be more frequently used by children aged between 4 and 4½. Children who made a single error in word meaning (semantic error) but who demonstrated full grammatical comprehension of a grammatically complex sentence were categorized by Marinac and Ozanne as using the semantic probability strategy. For example, a child who responded to 'Which red pencil has not been put away?' by indicating a blue pencil that had not been put away was considered to be using this strategy.

Comprehension strategies continue to be used by children when encountering more complex and less familiar grammatical structures (Tager-Flusberg 1989). Languages of the world differ significantly in how their grammars work – English relies mostly on word order to specify roles such as who did what to whom. Languages such as Hebrew, Turkish and Japanese rely more on morphemes – linguistic units that have meanings – to specify different grammatical roles, and have freer word order. This has implications for how children interpret grammatically more complex sentences – they tend to interpret them by adopting a strategy that makes use of the main way the grammar of their language works. For English-speaking 3- and 4-year-olds, this means interpreting a *passive* sentence such as 'The man was kissed by the woman' as an *active* sentence, 'The man kissed the woman'. These children are using a word-order strategy which involves ignoring the 'was' and 'by' and applying a generalized grammatical rule that the noun before the verb in a sentence corresponds to the person or thing that performs some action (the verb), and that the noun after the verb corresponds to the person or thing that has been affected by the action in some way (Bever 1970, discussed by Tager-Flusberg 1989).

Developments in verbal understanding

By the time children are 4 years old they are able to understand sentences with up to six separate pieces of information, and so are able to follow and participate in many different conversations, and understand long classroom instructions such as 'Get a thick green crayon from the small yellow box and give it to Sarah.' At 3½, children can often respond appropriately to 'How' questions such as 'How did you make the biscuits?', and towards the end of the fifth year they are able to understand 'When' questions such as 'When did you make the biscuits?' (James 1990, in Paul 1995). By the time they are 5, children can follow stories and respond appropriately to complex questions like 'What would we do if there were no houses?' They understand a vast range of different types of words – adjectives, prepositions, pronouns and negative terms.

By the age of 4, children are able to understand all basic grammatical structures but will continue to have difficulty working out the meaning of less common and more complex structures such as passive sentences and *relative clauses* (Tager-Flusberg 1989).

Understanding passive sentences

Towards the end of the fifth year, English-speaking children are able to understand passive sentences, providing the verb involves action of some sort (hit, jump, push, kiss) as in, 'The dog was hit by the man'; 'The boy was kissed by the girl'; 'The bike was pushed by the car' (Maratsos, Kucazj, Fox and Chalkley 1979, cited by Tager-Flusberg 1989). If the verb is a non-action verb, specifying an emotional or psychological state such as 'like', 'love', 'remember', 'think', then full comprehension does not occur until approximately 6 or 7.

Understanding relative clauses

Relative clauses are used to provide greater specification and thus differentiation to what a person is talking about. 'The man who is wearing a hat is climbing the tree', and 'The man is climbing the tree that towers above the house' are both more informative than 'The man is climbing the tree'. The first sentence contains a relative clause that specifies information about the man, while the second sentence contains a relative clause that specifies information about the tree. Most research looking at 4-year-old children's understanding of these types of sentences conclude that knowledge of the structures is incomplete, but that understanding of relative clauses that occur at the end of sentences precedes understanding of relative clauses that occur at the beginning or middle of sentences (Tager-Flusberg 1989). Children's understanding of relative clauses continues into the school years.

Understanding classroom language

As children move up the school from nursery onwards, they need to develop a good understanding of a range of basic linguistic concepts including those related to space (for example, above, below, behind, in front), quantity (for example, some, few, all), sequential ordering and time (for example, first, then, last, end, when, before, after), inclusion/exclusion (for example, one, either/or, but not, or, either) and *coordination* (for example, and, because). Understanding these types of words will enable children to:

- follow teachers' spoken instructions – 'Can all the boys stand in front of their chairs and all the girls stand behind theirs'
- develop literacy and numeracy skills – 'Which word ends in the letter p?', 'Who has got the most buttons?'
- participate in activities involving reasoning – 'Find all the pieces of fruit and place them in the red basket'
- express relationships between people, events and objects in their world – 'I want the one in the middle, please'.

Many children starting nursery have already learned the meanings of many of these words, and their knowledge and understanding of these types of words continues to develop as they get older (Boehm 2000). Developing knowledge and learning vocabulary, being able to follow what teachers say and the development of reading and writing skills all depend on a good understanding of these linguistic concepts.

Further developments in communication and expressive skills

The role of conversation in language learning

As children continue to develop over their fourth and fifth years, a significant increase is seen not only in the range of grammatical structures they are able to use but also in the range of communicative intentions, or functions, they are able to convey. Children need to test out their understanding of the grammatical structures they are acquiring, and need communicative contexts in which to do so (Dore 1979). Such a context is provided by conversation, which also provides:

- a rich source of grammatical structures
- a communicative context with plentiful opportunities for the child to interpret others' intentions

- a communicative context with opportunities for children to express a range of intentions through trying out different words and grammatical structures
- immediate feedback on the effectiveness of the message conveyed.

Children at this stage have come a long way from using a single sound or word to express a range of functions. Their gradual mastery of grammatical structures enables them to express a single function through various forms.

Example 4.2 Different grammatical structures express a single message

Three-year-old Cheyenne persisted in enticing her uncle to play with her, demonstrated in the three different types of sentence she uses to express the same intention. The intention she is conveying can be paraphrased as 'Please play hide and seek with me.'

CHEYENNE: Come on, come on . . . I need you . . . I need you . . . play hide and seek.
UNCLE: Oh, I can't play hide and seek before I have my coffee.
CHEYENNE: Well, we gotta go play, you see.
UNCLE: Play, yeah . . . Can't play without coffee.
CHEYENNE: Can you play hide and seek!

Cheyenne uses increasingly powerful and direct methods of engaging her uncle in the conversation in Example 4.2. She starts by stating what she wants her uncle to do ('I need you . . . I need you . . . play hide and seek'); when this fails she attempts to convince him that he does not have a choice in the matter ('Well we gotta go play, you see.'); after she still has not succeeded in getting her uncle to play with her, she resorts to asking a direct question ('Can you play hide and seek?'). It is not clear from making a purely linguistic analysis of the words used in this conversation whether Cheyenne is requesting information on the level of her uncle's skill in playing the game, or whether she is requesting his action. However, her intonation clearly conveyed that she was persisting in her attempts to get him to play with her. Cheyenne uses a range of grammatical structures, some of which she is still in the process of acquiring, in order to express the same underlying intention. Respectively, she attempts a complex sentence structure with *subordinate clause*, a future verb form and a direct *Yes–No question* form.

It is clear from listening to children talking at this stage that they have developed a very good understanding of what can be achieved through conversation (Dore 1979):

- conversation is a tool for achieving interactions with others, including peers, parents, teachers and other adults
- conversation supports the achievement of tasks through social negotiation and shared interaction.

Dore describes how nursery school children use conversation to provide the necessary stages of introducing and accomplishing tasks such as cleaning up after a painting session. Conversation serves to clarify and make explicit the sequence of steps necessary to planning and achieving a task. Example 4.3 contains a conversation among a group of preschool children who use language in various ways while preparing to play a game together.

Conversation skills development

Turn-taking

Children's abilities to hold conversations progress in that they are able to hold longer conversations and take longer turns, including on topics initiated by another person. Around the age of 4 they develop control over devices, such as repeating 'and . . .' to indicate they have not yet finished speaking (Pan and Snow 1999). They use not only pauses as cues to take turns in conversations, but also become sensitive to likely completion points as others are speaking, taking turns at appropriate linguistic junctures (Brinton and Fujuki 1989). They also become able to finish another speaker's turn if that speaker is unable to do so. Children have learned that they need to be persistent in order to enter a conversation, and that attention getting devices such as calling the listener's name assist in involving others in talk. The most successful devices used by 4-year-olds to enter or stay in conversations with peers are staying close to the speaker and maintaining eye contact.

Repairing conversations

After the age of 3, children start to initiate requests for clarification more, though even by the time they have entered school, most do not request clarification consistently when they have not understood what they hear (Pan and Snow 1999). It can be hard to encourage children to seek clarification under these circumstances, especially from adults, as they may be reluctant to question adults about things they have not understood (Brinton and Fujuki 1989).

Taking the listener's perspective

Over these years, children become better at gauging different listeners' needs for background information during conversation but may remain inconsistent in appropriate use of the relevant linguistic devices (Pan and Snow 1999). When giving an explanation of something that happened in the past involving other people and objects, for example, children may be inconsistent in using the people's or objects' names when introducing them, and may only use pronouns. In the following explanation the listener would have to ask several questions to clarify various elements: 'He put it on my one and I gave it back to him but . . . then I pushed him.'

Example 4.3 Preschool children's conversation supports interactive play

Conversation is used between 3-year-old twins Cheyenne and Alana, their 4-year-old sister Marnie and 2-year-old brother Tom, and an adult, during the course of a fishing game to variously announce intentions to play, explain rules of the game, seek confirmation that a fact has been understood, make descriptions, state facts, taunt, repair the game when it breaks down, seek permission to have a turn, regulate the flow of activity and turns, protest, seek information and state desires. Conversation thus provides a structure to the activity and facilitates the necessary stages involved for successful accomplishment of the game.

MARNIE:	Play fishing now.
ADULT:	How do you play?
ALANA:	You do this. *(demonstrates hooking a cardboard fish with a magnetic fishing rod)*
MARNIE:	You remember now, don't you?
CHEYENNE:	This all tangled. *(handling her fishing rod)*
ALANA:	*(sing-song intonation)* I got Cheyenne's fish! I got your fish!
CHEYENNE:	I need that one!
MARNIE:	I gonna get your fish! . . . I got it!
TOM:	Fish!
ADULT:	Fish! Tom's got a fish.
MARNIE:	Yeah, that's cheating . . . You haven't turned it on.
ALANA:	Can I catch this one?
ADULT:	Wait, Alana.
ALANA:	It's your go now.
MARNIE:	I didn't catch this one yet . . . Yeah, and after Alana, it's my go right?
ADULT:	That's right.
CHEYENNE:	Get again! Get the fish! Get the fish!
ALANA:	Oh, I don't want that one . . . No, Cheyenne, not your go.
ADULT:	What've you got, Cheyenne?
CHEYENNE:	It's a orange. *(orange fish)*
MARNIE:	I don't want to have a go. *(hits Tom)*

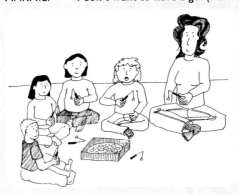

Figure 4.2 Preschool children using conversation

Around the age of 5 children use *articles* (a, an, the) more accurately when introducing new information (a, an) and when referring back to previously introduced information (the) (Pan and Snow 1999).

The topic of conversation

Children continue to rely largely on objects and events in the immediate environment as topics for striking up conversations. Adults continue to expand on topics introduced by children by alluding to topics drawn from past and future events (Brinton and Fujuki 1989). As they mature, children come to talk increasingly about ideas they have and become better at expressing alternative stances through role play and hypothesizing about possible future events (Pan and Snow 1999). They use a variety of nonlinguistic means (different voices, exaggerated use of eye gaze and intonation) to signal shifts between the real world and the pretend world (Pan and Snow 1999).

Uses of language

In addition to providing a context for the development of grammatical structures, conversation also supports the development of vocabulary and the use of language.

Children come to use their language skills for an increasingly wide range of purposes, as illustrated in Table 4.1. Two significant uses of language over the course of the fourth and fifth years are developments in the intellectual use of language and in the narrative genre, each of which is outlined below.

Intellectual use of language

Cooper *et al.* (1978) discuss the function of language as an intellectual process that assists in planning, guiding and integrating practical activities. This process occurs increasingly in an interactive context as outlined on pages 131–133. Conversations held by nursery-age children are seen by Dore (1979) to provide the context for participants to state their desires, beliefs and expectations as well as making explicit the various stages in individuals' schemes for accomplishing a goal. Over the course of the preschool years, self-monitoring by saying aloud the directions involved in accomplishing a task becomes so integral to how children function that directions eventually cease to be spoken aloud (Cooper *et al.* 1978). Children will continue to use externalized language when working out particularly difficult tasks (as do some adults), but directive language becomes internalized for more familiar or easier tasks, so that performance does not depend on the actual speaking of the words.

The development of narrative skills

Stories, or narratives, involving description of past events, become a regular part of children's conversations. Bruner (1990) describes how narrative helps organize

Table 4.1 Uses of language emerging between 3 and 5 years of age

Language use	Example
Requesting information or action	
Request for information	What's this?
Request for explanation	Why he go there?
Request for permission	Can I have one?
Request for action	Give me juice please.
Suggestions for action	Let's go downstairs.
Regulating conversation	
Initiates conversation	Hi! Hello! Mummy!
Requests clarification	Huh? What?
Identifies other as next speaker/player	Mummy? Marnie's go.
Identifies self as next speaker/player	You know what? My go.
Indicates openings, closings and shifts in conversation through use of boundary markers	Hi! Bye! Never mind. All right. By the way.
Uses politeness markers	Please. Thank you.
Statements of fact, rules, plans and internal states	
Labels objects, events and people	That's my mummy! That's your dinner.
Describes objects, events and people	I'm little. That's daddy's car.
Expresses emotions, intentions, beliefs, and desires	I'm sad. I'm gonna eat you up. I know that one. Now I'll draw mummy.
Expresses beliefs about another person's emotions, intentions, beliefs and desires	He want to see her. He's sad now. Daddy's gonna get me.
Makes judgments and expresses attitudes	You a good girl. You clever woman.
States rules and procedures, including social rules	You can't put it there. We not allowed to fight. No hitting. First bathtime, then story.
Gives explanations	Mummy's getting dressed cos she's going to work now.
Effects change in listener's state or knowledge	
States incongruous information for humorous effect	(Holding a strawberry) That's a lemon! No . . . that's a bean . . . not a strawberry!
Teases or playfully taunts listener	I'm gonna get you. You silly . . . billy!
Protests against hearer's behaviour	Stop singing! You don't say that one.
Warns against impending harm	Watch out! There is a monster coming!
Provides acknowledgements and answers	
Responds to *Yes–No* questions	Yes. No.
Answers to Wh- questions	It's a doggie. The monster's coming. I'm up here. I'm not doing nothing.
Agrees or disagrees	I'm not a big girl – I'm a little girl!
Acknowledges speaker's utterance	Yeah. Mmm. Oh.
Conveys attitudes or repeats others	
Makes exclamations to express surprise, delight and other attitudes	Oh! Wow! Yuck!
Repeats prior utterances	

Source: Adapted from Dore (1979), with permission of Academic Press.

our experiences. Our recollections of these, together with our impressions of the world, are formed into tales that we must keep recounting. Narrative acquisition is closely related to the ability to sequence information in a logical order and to organize that information into episodes. Component episodes, or story structure elements, of a narrative (adapted from Allen *et al.* 1994) include:

- *Settings* Introductions of the character/s, the location and time.
- *Initiating events* Occurrences that cause the character/s to act.
- *Internal responses* Goals, thoughts and feelings of the character/s.
- *Plans* Outline of the character/s' intended action/s.
- *Attempts* Actions undertaken by character/s in order to achieve goal/s.
- *Consequences* Success or failure of character/s in achieving goal/s. Effects of preceeding causes.

Children become able to tell about their own experiences as well as imaginary events. Narrative skills develop in the following sequence (adapted from Paul 1995, who acknowledges Applebee 1978, and Liles 1993):

- *Three years of age* Children tell short stories which consist of labelling events around a central character, event or theme. They might describe what characters have done; they might provide limited background information that helps the listener understand the story.

Example 4.4 Narratives of a 3½-year-old

At 3½, Elizabeth told the following stories about her experiences:

- 'I went to the seaside. I went in a boat. I fell down in the boat.'

- 'I went to a zoo. I went on a trip to see a monkey then I went to another zoo.'

- 'The Christmas fell down. I didn't have no Christmas. I did a Christmas with my dad. I put some Christmas tree.'

- 'I went to the football pitch. I played football. I tripped over. I felled and then blood was coming. Then I was starting to cry. My brother was in the football pitch. The ball was tripped me over.'

- *Four years of age* Stories are longer and have a central person, object or event. Children usually introduce the story, give background information, say what happened as the main event and how the story ended.

Example 4.5 Narratives of a 4½-year-old

At 4½, Jamie told this story as she was drawing a picture:

'A man lives in the house . . . a very old man with a very old lady and he can't get up but the lady helps him up. Just gets him up stairs with his wheelchair.'

She then told this story about her own experiences:

'A long time ago I went to the seaside and I got dressed and I went to the seaside with my dad. I couldn't . . . I got stuck in a big big hole and then my daddy picked me up. Then I went back home 'cos I was too cold.'

• *Five years of age* More information on the story setting is provided, with some evidence of cause–effect and temporal relations. Story endings may be abrupt and not always follow logically from the sequence of events so far, but often include an evaluation of the event in terms of how characters felt or what their intentions were.

Example 4.6 Narrative of a 5-year-old (Jessica)

At 5 years of age, Jessica told a story about a recent experience:

'My mummy took a photograph of me. Yesterday on Monday when there was no school. I smiled. Then I took the photograph home then my mummy cut one then my mummy put it in the photograph book of when I was a baby. Now I'm a grown up. I need the photograph to go to Spain because to let me in . . . in the plane. My mum's gonna put a photograph in the book . . . afterwards she's gonna show it to the man.'

Example 4.7 Narrative of a 5-year-old (Orla)

Also aged 5, Orla told the following story, which she subsequently called 'The funny daffodil':

'A princess was walking, okay? And there was, and on spring there was daffodils, okay? And there was all yellow daffodils and there was one red daffodil, okay? And a princess came along and it picked a red daffodil with all the other red daffodils, okay? And she put it in some water and then she took it out and then she got married.'

Example 4.8 Narrative of a 5-year-old (Matthew)

Matthew told the following version of a well-known story at the age of 5:

'I'll tell the three little pigs. The three little, the mummy said they have to leave at the house and then the three little pigs, the mummy said 'Take lots of healthy food, and keep your eyes open for the big wolf'. And then the little pig was stopping at for a break then he builded it with straw . . . the house. And then, and then, and then he the second little pig went to build it with wood and the big bad wolf still blowed it down and the third little pig build it with rocks and then 'Let me in, let me in'. And then he said, 'If you don't let me I'll puff and I'll blow your house down'. That's the end.'

Developments in expressive language structures

Linking ideas together and forming complex sentences

After children produce utterances that contain four or more words, they are ready to use complex sentences in order to express two or more ideas. This stage usually occurs towards the end of the third year, or early on in the fourth year. Complex sentences contain more than one verb and are first formed with conjunctions. Order of acquisition of conjunctions is: 'and', 'because', 'what', 'when', 'but', 'that', 'if' and 'so', with the use of 'and' decreasing as the other words are learned (Cooke and Williams 1985). Coordinating conjunctions (for example, and, because) are used to link ideas whose meanings would be equally clear if they were to stand on their own (see Example 4.9).

Other ways that children increase the length of their utterances is by linking two separate events within an utterance, and linking two separate factors within a single event (Cooke and Williams 1985). The meaning of the utterance depends on the expression of two or more factors or events, as illustrated in Examples 4.10 and 4.11. Both of these developments occur after children have started linking utterances through coordinating conjunctions; most children produce all types of complex sentences by their fourth birthdays (Mogford and Bishop 1993a).

Further developments in grammar in the fourth year

Over the fourth year children's utterances become increasingly grammatically correct and by their fourth birthday almost all basic grammatical structures will have been mastered (Bates *et al.* in press). This does not preclude production of grammatical errors, however, which may continue for another couple of years or so. Table 4.2 outlines the main developments in grammar over this period. It is important to view Table 4.2 as a general guide, given the great variability among children regarding acquisition of language structures.

Example 4.9 Using conjunctions in early complex sentences

Alana has begun to use complex sentences – linking together two or more ideas in an utterance with a coordinating conjunction, thus doubling the length of utterances:

ALANA: What's that?
ADULT: A tape recorder.
ALANA: Are you going to keep it?
ADULT: It's not mine – it's your dad's.
ALANA: Yeah – *it's my dad's and this one is mine* (indicating a video).

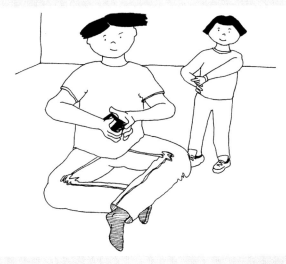

Figure 4.3 Three-year-old Alana discussing a tape recorder with her uncle

Children may use early conjunctions frequently, including when they are not strictly necessary or appropriate, as Cheyenne does in the following conversation.

CHEYENNE: This is my ears . . . 'cos I'm a panda, look!
ADULT: You're a panda?
CHEYENNE: Look, 'cos it's got ears. *(showing a picture of a panda)*
ADULT: It has, hasn't it.
CHEYENNE: 'Cos I'm a pan . . . 'cos it's a bear.

Example 4.10 Linking two events in complex sentences

Complex sentences – linking two separate events within an utterance, where the meaning of the utterance depends on the expression of both events:

- My mummy's gonna get me sweeties when she goes shopping.
- We can play hide and seek as soon as we get home.

Example 4.11 Linking two separate factors in complex sentences

Complex sentences – linking two separate factors within a single event:

- Mummy made me cry.
- Monsters make me run away.

Further developments in grammar in the fifth year and later

It has been suggested by Karmiloff-Smith (in Bates *et al.* in press) that between the ages of 4 and 6, the way that grammar is used by children undergoes significant changes, from a single sentence level to a discourse- or text-level, as in the narrative genre, involving decontextualized use of language. For example, correct use of pronouns and articles (i.e. a, an or the) depend on prior introduction of elements into a conversation or written text and thus provide linguistic cohesion. Mogford and Bishop (1993a) illustrate the importance of these devices in two versions of the same short story; in the first version they are absent, while in the second some are present:

First version: a boy went in a garden
a boy met a monster
a monster ate up a boy

Second version: a boy went into the garden
he met a monster
the monster ate him up

Selection of correct devices such as articles and pronouns depends not only on the ability to sequence events correctly, but also on making accurate assumptions about what the listener or reader already knows or does not know. Correct use of grammar, then, is interwoven inextricably with pragmatic knowledge. As has already been discussed previously in this chapter, the narrative genre is encountered increasingly as children move up the school system.

Table 4.2 Common features of grammatical development between 3 and 5 years of age

Grammatical structure	Examples
Pronouns	
I, you, he, she, we, they	You give me that one.
	They are Dad's. Can we have biscuits?
Prepositions	
Under, behind, in front of, beside, next to	It's behind you! Sit next to me.
Verbs	
Can, will, is, are, am, have, do	She can reach the book.
used correctly on most occasions by 5,	They're going to crash
including to express past and future	He's spilt his milk. He'll fall in.
Verb tenses are marked:	
irregular past,	We went to the zoo.
Regular past and future	Joey stopped playing. We'll all eat together.
Questions	
Using can, will, is, are, am, have, do	Will you help me? Can I have some?
Reversing the order of the verb and noun	What are you doing? Where is daddy going?
Why? (predominates at 4)	Why is the baby small?
How? when? (later)	When is Grandma coming?
Tag questions	Daddy's coming home, isn't he?
Negatives	
By 42 months doesn't, isn't are used	She doesn't want to sleep! It isn't there.
By 4, didn't, couldn't, wasn't are used	She didn't wash her hair. Mum couldn't find her keys. There wasn't a monkey.
After 4 years, nobody, none, nothing	There's nothing in my bag.
and no one are used	I'm not doing nothing.

Sources: Tager-Flusberg (1989) and Brown (1973).

Bates *et al.* (in press) suggest that any further developments in grammar that occur after the age of 4, such as the correct use of passive sentences, are likely to occur gradually over the forthcoming years.

Errors that children make in their fourth and fifth years

Despite having grasped the major grammatical structures and having at their disposal vocabularies that number thousands of words during these years, it is still very common for children to make grammatical errors. For example, gender errors are common when using pronouns up to the age of 4, resulting in sentences like, 'Give it to my daddy – put it on her head!' Grammatical rules may be over-generalized, as in application of the '-ed' past tense ending to irregular past tense forms – 'I putted it on the table'. It may take some time before children can correctly distinguish *mass* and *count nouns*, producing expressions like, 'I'm watching a sky'. Generally, grammatical errors such as these are signs that children are trying to work out general rules that can be applied to words in a certain grammatical context, and are therefore a good sign. Grammatical errors may continue to occur for a couple more years or so.

Speech development

Main features of speech development

By the age of 4½ a child's pronunciation closely resembles that of an adult. While many children in their fourth year will continue to use some simplification patterns (see pages 75–77 and 112–114 for a discussion of simplification patterns), many of these, if not all, have disappeared by a child's fourth birthday (Grunwell 1987). This progression towards a more mature, adult type pronunciation pattern results from a combination of:

- increasing awareness of the discrepancies between immature pronunciations and adult pronunciations
- motivation to make changes to one's own speech
- knowing how to articulate the full range of speech sounds, in all positions of words
- developments in the child's motor speech control, resulting in a more appropriate rate of speech and greater consistency in pronunciation of words.

(Hewlett 1990)

Table 4.3 specifies simplification patterns that can persist through these years. Over the first half of the fourth year, children learn to produce some blends such as 'tr' in 'train', 'cl' in 'clean', 'gr' in 'green, 'sn' in 'snow', 'mp' in 'jump' and 'nt' in 'went' (Grunwell 1987). They still have difficulty producing sounds that are complicated to articulate and/or that are confusing perceptually at this age, such as 'ch', 'j', 'sh', 'z' ,'v', 'th', 'f', 'r' and 'w', but have usually started to pronounce these half-way through the fifth year (Cooke and Williams 1985, Stackhouse and Wells 1997).

Table 4.3 Examples of speech simplification processes that might persist through the fourth and fifth years

Target word	Child's pronunciation	Simplification process
tomato	mato	weak syllable deletion
stop	top	's' blend reduction
crisps	kips	reduction of blends other than 's'
never, then	neder, den	stopping
thankyou, ship	fankyou, sip	fronting
peach, sandwich	peats, sandwids	fronting
run, yellow	wun, lellow	gliding

Table 4.4 illustrates the gradual nature of pronunciation development over the early years, and is based on Grunwell's (1987: 231) 'Profile of Phonological Development'. There is increasing complexity in pronunciation through the years as more sounds and syllable patterns are acquired. It is important to treat the age levels as general guidelines only, given the wide variation that exists among children regarding speech development. When reading the child's pronunciations in Table 4.4, say them as they are written.

Table 4.4 Chronological profile of pronunciation ability

Approximate age	Pick	Tomato sandwich	Christmas tree
18–24 months	bi	mado bambi	didma dee
24–30 months	bi	mado damwi	didma dee
30–36 months	pik	mato tamwid	kitmat tee
36–42 months		mato samwidz	kwismas twee
42–54 months		mato samwidge	kwismas twee
54 months +		tomato samwidge	krismas tree

Developmental dysfluency

It is not uncommon for children in their fourth or fifth year (and sometimes earlier) to experience disruptions to the normal flow of speech. Stackhouse and Wells (1997) and Bernstein Ratner (1989) characterize dysfluent speech in the following ways:

- a greater number of hesitations
- repetitions of words, sounds or syllables
- rephrasing of utterances
- use of fillers such as 'um' and 'well' between words
- struggles to make correct word choices.

Dysfluency might emerge around the time that a child is achieving major linguistic developments such as complex sentence production. More grammatically complex phrases and sentences are harder for children to plan. This can pose a significant challenge to the child's developing ability to integrate the various aspects of speech production and language formulation (Bernstein Ratner 1989, Stackhouse and Wells 1997). Most children pass through a stage of dysfluency as part of normal speech and language development. A proportion of children will develop stammering, when dysfluent speech interferes with communicating and causes distress to the speaker or listener.

Emergent literacy skills

Preschool children develop knowledge about the uses and nature of written language long before they are able to decode or manipulate letters – this knowledge is referred to as emergent literacy (Dickinson *et al.* 1989, Paul 1995).

Factors affecting emergent literacy skills

Children who grow up in homes where book sharing is encouraged are more likely to develop emotional bonds to books and an expectation to become literate. They will also have opportunities to become familiar with the genre of literary language which involves more precise and abstract vocabulary, more complex grammar and a wider range of uses of language than usually occurs in spoken language (Paul 1995). Each of these factors has been found to support the move towards full literacy (Dickinson *et al.* 1989, Paul 1995).

Characteristics of emergent literacy skills

Dickinson *et al.* (1989) support Lomax and McGee's claim that the progression of emergent literacy skills follows a hierarchical pattern. Initially children develop concepts of what books are – what they look like, where they are kept, what they feel like and how they are used – followed by a developing awareness of the purpose of print. The child comes to learn that, if she covers up the black squiggles on the page while her caregiver is reading a story, it is not until she removes her hand that the adult can resume telling the story. The child begins to learn that the black squiggles hold some meaning. They pretend to 'read' books, using appropriate intonation and supplying correct words now and again. Children draw adults' attention to environmental print, such as street signs and shop names, and food packaging labels. In their fourth year, children begin to show interest in rhyming and *alliteration*, both of which are to do with analysing words into their component parts (syllables and sounds respectively) and which lay the foundations for later literacy skills.

Links between spoken and written language skills

Narrative

There is strong agreement among developmental language and literacy researchers that spoken language skills lay the foundations for literacy to develop. If children have restricted understanding or use of spoken vocabulary, continue to rely on non-linguistic comprehension strategies and have poor understanding of the grammatical structures that occur in decontextualized language, they will have difficulty comprehending narratives, regardless of whether the narrative is spoken or written (Paul 1995).

Phonological awareness

Speech sound awareness, or phonological awareness, refers to the conscious awareness of the sounds of a language. It is the ability to manipulate and reflect on the sounds in words separate to the meanings of words. Producing and understanding speech are automatic processes, with no need to attend consciously to the speech sounds. An *alphabetic* writing system, however, demands explicit awareness of speech sounds. Paul (1995), Catts and Vartiainen (1993) and Stackhouse and Wells (1997) describe phonological awareness as:

- the awareness of aspects such as the length of syllables or words
- the awareness of rhyming properties of words and that words may begin or end with the same sound (as in the game 'I spy')
- analytical knowledge that enables words to be broken down into component syllables or sounds (for spelling), to understand that sounds can be represented by letters, to learn the sound–letter correspondence rules and to blend sounds represented by letters into words (for reading).

There is much evidence to suggest that there are close links between speech, language, phonological awareness and literacy abilities in children (Paul 1995, Stackhouse and Wells 1997). Paul (1995) cites studies by various researchers that have shown phonological awareness to be the best predictor in reading ability. She also cites Webster and Plante 1992, who have suggested that children's skills in phonological awareness depend, at least in part, on their language abilities. These skills generally start to emerge over the course of a child's fourth year. Table 4.5, which draws on work by Paul (1995), outlines the chronological development of phonological awareness skills over the fourth and fifth years.

Table 4.5 Chronological development of phonological awareness skills

Skill	Example
Rhyming	You *silly billy willy*
Segmenting words into syllables	Give me a banana…*ba-na-na…ba–na–na*
Identifying words with same first sound	*Milly* and *Molly* and *mop* and *moo-cow*
Identifying words with same last sound	*pin* and *hen* and *gone* and *in*
Counting sounds in words and	'hen' has three sounds – *h…eh…n*
Segmenting simple words into sounds	'up' has two sounds – *uh…p*
Segmenting words with consonant blends into sounds	'trip' has four sounds – *t…r…i…p*
	'paste' has four sounds – *p…ay…s…t*
	'crisp' has five sounds – *k…r…i…s…p*
Manipulating sounds in words	What's left if we take 'g' from 'gone'? – '*on*'
	What word do we make if we swop the first and last sounds of 'peach'? – '*cheap*'

Source: Paul (1995).

Summary of Chapter 4

Attention control

1 In the fourth year children are able to spontaneously shift their focus of attention from what they are currently engaged in to what a speaker is saying without needing adult prompting and in the fifth year they develop integrated attention. This means they are able to learn in a classroom where instructions are given while children are currently engaged in an activity.

Links between play and language

2 Children's pretend play during the fourth and fifth years:

- reflects their growing understanding of the world, and in particular of social relationships
- illustrates their ability to distinguish between reality and pretend, and thus to appreciate that there are different mental representations of the world
- becomes increasingly linked to positive and effective social interaction and communication skills
- is closely linked to the development of narrative skills, which is in turn a fundamental feature of written language and thus a key to school achievement.

3 Parents who mediate children's viewing of television programmes and videos can use these as a basis for interaction, conversation and related activities. High levels of television viewing is speculated to have a negative impact on children's attention and language development.

Semantic and vocabulary development

4 By the time they are 5, children understand thousands of words and start to define words according to function properties. Expressive vocabulary is also extensive.

Understanding words and sentences

5 By the age of 4, children understand most basic grammatical structures; acquisition of more complex structures continues in to the school years, and is reflected in the continued use of some comprehension strategies. Five-year-olds no longer need pictures in order to understand stories.

Further developments in communication and expressive skills

6 By the time they are 5, children:

- are able to use their communication skills for an increasingly wide range of social and intellectual purposes
- are able to express an underlying intention through a range of grammatical structures
- can engage in conversations that last a number of turns around an established topic
- can tell short stories that contain an appropriate amount of information, that include a beginning, middle and end, and that might include some description or evaluation of the situation.

7 Conversation provides a context for children to practise their developing expressive language skills, and for them to use language for different purposes.

8 Children come to use all basic grammatical structures over the fourth and fifth years; significantly they start to use complex sentences consisting of more than one main idea – consequently utterances are longer.

Speech development

9 While some simplification patterns may still be used, children's pronunciation is generally clear by the age of 4½.

Emergent literacy skills

10 There is a close link between competence in spoken language and competence in development of literacy skills.

11 Phonological awareness skills, which underlie literacy development, emerge in the fourth year.

Key skills 4.1 Communication skills usually achieved by 4-year-old children

- Seeks out and enjoys companionship of peers
- Engages in dramatic make-believe play with peers
- Holds conversation skilfully with a variety of people
- Able to shift attention spontaneously from what she is doing to what somebody is saying and back to what she is doing again
- Continues to use strategy of doing what is usually done in response to improbable instructions (for example 'Make the baby feed mum')
- Understands sentences with up to six key words (for example 'Put the *small bag* and the *cup under Daddy's chair*')
- Understands and uses all basic grammatical structures, with occasional mistakes (for example 'I went to the circus and sawed the clowns')
- Uses language to express ideas and feelings, discuss plans, problem-solve and negotiate
- Asks lots of questions, especially using 'How?' and 'Why?'
- Able to express herself clearly on most occasions, reflecting a vocabulary consisting of thousands of words
- Uses complex sentences with two or more verbs to link ideas
- Tells stories about connected past events providing:

  - an introduction, sufficient background knowledge, account of what happened
  - information on how the story ended

- Uses 'can', 'will', 'is', 'are', 'have', 'do' correctly (for example 'I can jump')
- Speech is clear, with few immaturities (for example, thank you → fank you)

Before using this table, see page xxi.

Key skills 4.2 Communication skills usually achieved by 5-year-old children

- Cooperative with peers, understanding the need for fair play
- Engages in dramatic make-believe play, particularly with peers
- Uses language as main means of communicating
- Holds conversation easily on a number of topics with a variety of people
- Shows mature attention and listening; can be taught in a classroom; easily integrates what somebody says with what she is doing
- Understands most grammatical structures; continuing to develop an understanding of more complex sentences (for example 'The cow was pushed by the horse', 'The boy who is standing next to the shortest girl is the one who's got all the biscuits')
- Understands and responds appropriately to 'How?' and 'Why?' questions
- Follows complicated stories without the need for pictures
- Able to express herself clearly on most occasions, reflecting a vocabulary that consists of thousands of words
- Able to define words according to function (for example, a car is for driving)
- Tells stories including an evaluation in terms of how characters felt or what their intentions were; starts to make predictions
- Uses pronouns and articles correctly when telling stories
- Starts to ask questions using 'When?'
- Continues to make grammatical errors (for example 'My feets are cold')
- Speech is clear to familiar and unfamiliar listeners; possible difficulty pronouncing 'th', 'ch', 'j', 'v'

Before using this table, see page xxi.

Warning signs 4.1 Possible warning signs for 4-year-old children

- Has difficulty or is uninterested in mixing or playing with peers
- Shows little imagination, especially in play
- Unable to concentrate on anything for longer than a few minutes at a time
- Unable to hold conversations easily about past and future events
- Frequently looks bemused when spoken to; does not carry out instructions
- Unable to give a clear account of events at which listener was not present
- Does not ask or respond appropriately to most 'Wh' questions (for example 'Where do we go shopping?', 'Who lives at home with you?')
- Only understands and uses a small vocabulary
- Uninterested in stories
- Does not show clear understanding of a range of concepts relating to size, shape, position, colour and quantity
- Does not use range of grammatical structures (for example, verb endings and plurals, as in 'Yesterday we picked flowers')
- Struggles to produce sentences and to get the words out
- Speech is very unclear
- Stammering
- Parents express concerns, are worried or anxious

⚠ Before using this table, see page xxii.

Warning signs 4.2 Possible warning signs for 5-year-old children

- **Unable to hold and understand normal conversation**
- **Easily distracted in the classroom**
- **Unusually withdrawn or disruptive**
- **Difficulty in organizing self and following classroom routine without copying peers**
- **Difficulty in attending to, understanding and remembering group instructions.**
- **Requires individual support to carry out instructions given to a group**
- **Uninterested in stories, or only focuses on details**
- **Responds better than others to visually oriented tasks**
- **Has poor understanding of concepts relating to size, shape, position, quantity and temporal ordering; poor sequencing skills**
- **Difficulty formulating phrases and sentences and relaying information verbally**
- **Difficulty giving coherent account of recent past experiences**
- **Difficulty finding the right words when speaking; may use words incorrectly or make up words**
- **Stammering**
- **Unclear speech – all sounds should be correct by the age of 6 or 7**
- **Difficulty generating rhymes or beating the number of syllables in a word**
- **Parents express concerns, are worried or anxious**

⚠ See below.

Warning signs 4.3 Absolute indicators for immediate evaluation

Filipek and Prizant (1999) produced the following set of warning signs. According to these writers, identification of any one of these signs indicates the need for immediate assessment of a child's communication skills development.

- **No warm, joyful engagement by five months (for example, no big smiles)**
- **No two-way, back-and-forth gesturing by nine months (for example, no smiles that encourage a smile, no sounds the encourage vocalization)**
- **No babbling by 12 months**
- **No pointing or other gestures by 12 months**
- **No single words by 16 months**
- **No two-word spontaneous (not copied) phrases by 24 months**
- **ANY loss of ANY language or babbling or social skills at ANY age**

⚠ Before using these tables, see page xxii.

Learning more than one language in early childhood

5

○ What is 'bilingualism'?
○ Stages and features of bilingual acquisition in children under 5 when learning two languages at the same time and at different times; introduction to the theories of bilingual acquisition.
○ Links between bilingualism, cognitive development and literacy development in early childhood.
○ Social and cultural aspects of growing up bilingual; environmental factors affecting bilingual acquisition and implications of these for supporting bilingual children at home and in education.
○ Summary of key points.

It is important to acknowledge that bilingualism is a huge topic to cover; the content of this chapter comprises some aspects that are fundamental to an understanding of what is involved when learning more than one language in early childhood. The terms 'bilingual' and 'bilingualism' refer to two languages; while it is acknowledged that many speakers use and/or understand more than two languages, these terms are used in this book when referring to the use and acquisition of more than one language, for purposes of clarity.

Bilingualism

Defining bilingualism

All speakers, whether *monolingual* or *bilingual*, are able to adapt their style of speaking in order to fulfill different purposes. Miller (1978) drew a link between monolingual speakers' ability to switch between different levels of formality in their use of words, grammar and pronunciation according to interaction variables such as the status of the speaker and the setting, and bilingual speakers' use of 'two interacting languages which complement each other'. For example, an adult speaker might conceivably say 'Pass the sugar' to a close friend but not to someone he did not know well. They might say, 'Could you possibly pass the sugar?' to less familiar adults.

Any definition of bilingualism needs to go beyond the individual speaker as its focus to take into account the speaker's circumstances, which include the social, cultural and linguistic contexts. Definitions of bilingualism over the years have focused on linguistic competence (for example Hall 1952, cited by Miller 1978: 19 – 'bilingualism does not begin until the speaker has at least some knowledge and control of the grammatical structures of the second language') and fluency (for example Bloomfield 1933, cited by Miller 1978: 18 – 'native like control of two languages'). Garcia (1982, in Malavé 1997) specifies that bilingual acquisition necessarily takes place during the first five years of life; that both comprehension and expressive skills are acquired; that learning occurs in a natural way through social interaction; and that learning of the two languages occurs simultaneously. Children from many ethnic minority communities in the UK, US and Australasia, however, whose families speak a *minority language*, are introduced to a *majority language* during the preschool years. Discussion of what is meant by the terms 'minority' and 'majority' languages can be found on page 155. Madhani (1994) suggests a useful and broad definition of bilingualism as 'understanding and using two or more languages to varying degrees at various times'. This definition can apply to an individual speaker and the wider community. It is important to note that 'use of language' can extend to include spoken and written language.

Bilingual communities and patterns of language use

The precise number of bilingual speakers worldwide is not known; however, Baker (1996) estimates that approximately two-thirds of the world speaks more than one language. In parts of Europe and south-eastern Asia speakers of the same language inhabit different but neighbouring countries, and within India and South Africa several distinct languages are spoken (Genesee 1993). In many parts of Africa, India, Asia and Europe bilingualism is commonplace, in contrast to the US and UK where monolingualism is generally perceived as the norm.

Children growing up in bilingual environments may find themselves in a range of different circumstances. These include intermarriage between speakers of different languages, socio-economic pressures for speakers to learn other languages for functional purposes such as securing work, and large-scale international migration which has resulted in minority language speakers in all parts of the world. There are as many different variations of language use among bilingual individuals as there are bilingual speakers. However, common patterns of language use have been identified for most bilingual speakers, albeit very roughly in many cases.

Patterns of language use in families of children who are bilingual from birth

Four patterns of language use among families who raise children bilingually from birth have been identified by Langdon and Cheng (1992):

- one person, one language (for example, mother speaks only Hebrew, father speaks only English to their child)
- one place, one language (for example, Hebrew spoken only at home and in other Hebrew-speaking homes, English spoken outside of the home)
- one time of day, one language (for example, both parents speak one language during the day, the other language in the evening and at night time)
- alternating use of both languages (for example, both parents switch between using both languages depending on contextual factors such as other people present, the topic, the location and the activity).

Each of these patterns appears to work well for children who have no difficulties with the development of their communication skills.

Patterns of language use in linguistic minority communities

Patterns of language use among minority language speakers, such as Bengali speakers in the UK, will be comparable between different established linguistic minority communities, regardless of the languages involved (Martin 1994). The heritage, or minority, language is used predominantly for matters pertaining to the family, social arrangements, the home, child rearing, caring and religious and cultural dealings. The dominant, or majority, language is used more when communicating outside of the linguistic minority community for all other aspects of living, such as education, health, employment, travel and shopping. There are of course differences among individuals regarding willingness, competence and ability to use the heritage and dominant languages.

The relationship between language use and language proficiency in bilingual speakers

Bilingualism is a relative phenomenon and bilingual speakers differ in the degree to which they are proficient in one language over another. Language proficiency is closely related to the speaker's pattern of language use in different contexts, such as the street, at school or at home (Baker 1996). Some speakers are equally proficient in both languages (*'balanced'* or *'productive' bilinguals*) while others retain a passive understanding of one language but use the other language in an active way for communication (*'passive' bilinguals*).

For purposes of clarity, the term 'minority language' is used in this book to refer to the language that an ethnic minority community uses at home, and 'majority language' refers to the language spoken by those in the wider community. For example, when considering the Bangladeshi community in the UK, Bengali would be the minority language, and English the majority language.

Most bilingual speakers have a stronger command over one of their languages at any one time (Watson 1995). Language '*dominance*' is used in this book to refer to relative levels of proficiency an individual has in each language. The dominant language is that which a speaker is more competent in using. When the wider linguistic environment changes, as can occur for example when visiting relatives in another country, or when a young child who has been looked after at home starts going to nursery, language dominance can also change fairly quickly (Watson 1995).

There is a relationship between language and power that has special implications for minority language speakers in the context of a majority culture. Higher levels of proficiency in the majority language increases access to education and employment, and leads to higher socio-economic status and wider social relations. This can have a significant impact on socio-cultural expectations within a family, and on the roles of different family members.

There can be significant differences between generations concerning patterns of language use and proficiency in both minority and majority languages, with first generation children of immigrants growing up with greater proficiency in the majority language, frequently at the expense of their minority language (Genesee 1993, Malavé 1997). Loss of the minority language can take place within two or three generations of immigration (Langdon and Cheng 1992) and is largely affected by how immigrants feel about the migration experience, the size of the ethnic community and integration to the majority culture through mixed marriages. Speakers' attitudes towards the languages they speak are strongly influenced by the relative status of each language and also impact on the maintenance of a lower status minority language (Hakuta and D'Andrea 1990). This *affective variable* was found to be a far stronger predictor of how Mexican children living in Northern California, USA, maintained Spanish than how quickly or proficiently they learned English. These factors are further discussed on pages 172–173.

Increasing bilingualism in western countries

All sources of evidence point towards increasing rates of bilingualism among families in western countries, largely due to patterns of migration. Children from linguistic minority backgrounds were estimated in 1999 to form roughly one-tenth of the pupil population in the UK (Crutchley 1999).

Less established minority language speakers, such as refugees, may exhibit differences in patterns of language use. Refugees, especially young children, might be reluctant to speak the majority language, for a variety of reasons including emotional trauma (Martin 1994).

It is important to conclude this section by noting that while bilingual speakers and communities demonstrate identifiable patterns of language use and that differences exist between speakers regarding language competence, each family has a unique profile of language history, of relationships to minority and majority cultures, of reasons and incentives for raising bilingual children and of patterns of language use (Watson 1995).

Features of bilingual speech and the patterns and stages of bilingual acquisition

Bilingual acquisition can be *simultaneous* or *sequential*. Simultaneous acquisition occurs when two languages are introduced at the same time in infancy; sequential acquisition occurs when one language is introduced after the child has developed a basic acquisition in their first language, which has usually taken place by the end of the third year. Each pattern has different implications for language development, which are discussed in the following pages. Before looking at the patterns of acquisition, however, it is useful to consider some of the features of bilingual speech in mature bilingual speakers, as these can influence the language development of bilingual children.

Features of bilingual speech

Code mixing and code switching

Bilingual adults commonly mix the languages they speak depending on a range of factors. Mixing occurs both within single utterances and over several turns in conversations (referred to as *code mixing* and *code switching* respectively), and might encompass all levels of language: speech sounds, vocabulary, grammar and type of message conveyed. Genesee (1993) cites studies of code switching in adults which reveal it to be a 'sophisticated, rule-governed communicative device used by linguistically competent bilinguals to achieve a variety of communicative goals, such as conveying emphasis, role playing, establishing socio-cultural identity'.

There is evidence (Poplack 1979, in Genesee) that code mixing and code switching increase as bilingual adults' competence in the two languages increases. Mixing occurs in response to subtle interaction and sociolinguistic factors such as the appropriate way of addressing another speaker, their ethnic and linguistic identity, and the setting, tone and purpose of the communication (Miller 1978, Genesee 1993). Bilingual children develop the conscious ability to distinguish between two language systems between the ages of 3 and 6 (Miller 1978). Prior to this age, bilingual children's mixing of languages is unsystematic, in contrast to mature bilingual speakers' mixing, which is systematic (Genesee 1993). The ability to reflect on language (*metalinguistic awareness*) at this early age is an advantage for bilingual children and is further discussed on pages 169–171.

A typical situation which gives rise to code mixing by competent bilingual adults is given in the following example. Parents of a child and teachers who are Yiddish/English-speakers from the same Orthodox Jewish minority community hold a meeting at the child's nursery. Many members of the Orthodox Jewish community speak Yiddish. This community has been well established in the majority English-speaking culture for several generations. Individuals from the majority English-speaking culture also attend the meeting, and most of the discussion is in English. This would normally be the case even in the absence of monolingual English-speakers, as English is the main language used in matters of education, and consequently many bilingual speakers have developed dominance in English to talk about such matters. Code mixing by the bilingual speakers takes place when the subject matter relates to cultural and religious issues particular to the Orthodox Jewish community, and therefore might include some Hebrew words. This is because several Hebrew words whose meanings relate to matters of religion are used by all Orthodox Jews, regardless of which language or languages they speak. Words which have strong religious significance, and which therefore sound most 'natural' to the speakers in Hebrew, are less likely to be spoken in English. This can result in utterances such as, 'We can help him do the actions to the brocha', where, although there is an English equivalent (brocha roughly translates as 'blessing'), the Hebrew word is the one of choice. An extended discussion around a topic of socio-cultural identity, and which naturally involves code switching between the bilingual teacher and parents in Yiddish, may then ensue.

Interference

The weaker language spoken by people who are bilingual is sometimes subject to an *interference effect* from the dominant language. This effect can occur at all levels of language – the sound of a foreign accent is due to phonological interference (the effect of the dominant language's speech sound system on that of the weaker speech sound system). Interference at the grammatical level can result in the sentence 'the dog eats the bone', for example, being produced by a Bengali/English-speaker as 'dog bone eats'. The speaker's dominant language is Bengali; differences between English and Bengali grammar result in the sentence being coded as 'dog bone eats'. Bengali rules regarding word order in sentence formation and use of the word 'the' affect production of the sentence in English. As all languages have unique sets of rules governing all levels of language, interference effects from one language onto another will differ according to which languages are involved.

Simultaneous acquisition of more than one language

Children acquiring two languages proceed through the same stages of language development as monolingual speakers learning the same language (Genesee 1993) and attain social interaction and receptive language milestones at similar times as monolingual speakers; expressive language milestones in bilingual children before the age of 3 should be extended by two or three months, however (Watson 1995, Watson and Cummins 1999). All children learning two languages simultaneously demonstrate errors in speech and language which are comparable to those errors of normal language development made by monolingual children. Mixing of two languages by bilingual learners might occur for words, grammatical structures, intonation and speech sounds from their two languages, and is further discussed in the following sections.

Different writers over the years have proposed different models of simultaneous bilingual acquisition, each with different implications for the underlying system, or systems, of language processing. Children approach the task of learning two languages simultaneously, with no fundamental differences in their cognitive abilities, knowledge of the world, social understanding or communicative competence from monolingual children of the same age (Genesee 1993). The fundamental questions raised are:

- Do these children start out with a *unitary language system* which encompasses both languages being acquired, and which then becomes differentiated at some stage after infancy?
- Alternatively, do they develop *differentiated language systems*, one for each language being learned, right from the start?

Each of these viewpoints is considered in the following pages. Although these are important theoretical considerations, it is important not to lose sight of the fact that both viewpoints lead towards childhood bilingualism.

From undifferentiated to differentiated language systems

Volterra and Taeschner (1978) proposed three stages, described below, that children learning two languages simultaneously may demonstrate in terms of how they select words and put them together.

STAGE 1

Words and the rules governing how words are ordered in sentences are unified in a single language system. Children are thought to have one mental 'dictionary' for vocabulary, rather than two separate ones. Children mix words from both languages when talking, as Andreu, a 1-year, 10-month-old Catalan/English-speaking boy does in the following example when talking with his father, who is holding a conversation with his son in English (Juan-Garau and Perez-Vidal 2001: 80) (translations into English are in brackets):

FATHER: Where's that teddy?
ANDREU: Aqui. *(pointing, 'here')*
FATHER: No, that's not the teddy, is it?

Andreu switches from understanding English to speaking in Spanish in the context of the conversation with his English-speaking father.

STAGE 2

Children start to develop two differentiated vocabulary systems for the relevant languages, but continue to mix the two languages' grammatical systems. If one language has an easier grammatical structure, it may appear dominant for a while. There is evidence to suggest that highly inflected languages (Turkish and Panjabi for example), as opposed to those which depend predominantly on word order to specify grammatical relations, are easier to learn. Developmental grammatical mixing results in utterances similar in type to those produced by mature bilingual speakers who experience an interference effect from their dominant language. Although the end results may resemble each other, the process underlying mixing in the young bilingual speaker who is developing language systems for two languages is distinct from that in the mature bilingual speaker, who has an established language system. Laura, who was learning English, French and Greek, had this conversation about her drawing with her French/English-speaking mother at the age of 2 years and 9 months (translations into English are in brackets):

LAURA: Ma p'tit mer à moi. *(My little sea.)*
MOTHER: C'est la petite mer à toi. *(That's your little sea.)*
LAURA: C'est Laura petit mer. *(That's Laura's little sea.)*

Although speaking French with her mother, Laura uses the English word order to express possession (Laura's little sea). Correct French grammar would necessitate the following word order: 'C'est la petite mer de Laura', i.e. 'Laura' should occur after 'petite mer'. (Laura makes additional errors in her utterances, which are not the subject of current inquiry.) Other examples of grammatical mixing by Laura on the same day are, 'la bébé mer' and 'mummy's mer' which, from the contexts, are interpreted as 'the baby's sea' and 'mummy's sea' respectively. 'Mummy's mer' provides an additional example of mixing the vocabularies of French and English (Laura made this utterance in response to her mother's question which was, that time, in English).

STAGE 3

The two languages become differentiated on all levels – vocabulary, grammatical rules, speech sounds and intonation. Young children may associate the two languages rigidly with people or settings and elect to speak a certain language only with particular adults and/or in particular locations. Children make normal developmental errors in both languages, and may over-use certain grammatical rules within languages in order to keep languages separate. For example, all adjectives are placed before the noun in English (a *chatty* girl) and most after the noun in French (une fille *bavarde*). Children are able to learn exceptions to these rules when they become more confident and flexible in each language (Watson 1995). Such an example in French is the phrase 'a big house', which is expressed by placing the word for 'big' – 'grande' – before the noun: 'une *grande* maison'.

Differentiated language systems from birth

Genesee (1993), however, questions the notion of a unified language system in the early stages of simultaneous bilingual acquisition and proposes that children are able to differentiate between language systems from the earliest stages of language development. Genesee cites studies that have shown infants in the first few weeks of life to show sensitivity towards small differences in speech sounds of languages they have never been exposed to, and 4-day-old infants from French-speaking families to differentiate between French and Russian, and to show a preference for French.

Genesee states that the role of linguistic input, in particular from parents, determines strongly the degree to which mixing between languages occurs in children's utterances. He states the importance of taking into account contextual factors when analysing bilingual children's utterances, and makes the observation that children mix languages more when their parents also mix languages when addressing them. Bilingual children are seen to be highly sensitive to the variables within interaction and, taking the adult's lead regarding language use (i.e. which language is spoken), adapt their language use accordingly. At the age of 2½, Laura and her native French-speaking mother, who had both recently returned to England from a trip to France, held the following conversation (translations into English are in brackets):

MOTHER: Chien jaune (yellow dog) . . . do you want to see the pictures?
LAURA: Oui. (Yes.)
MOTHER: Ah . . . va chercher les photos. (Go and get the photos.) *(Laura takes a packet of photos from a shelf and returns to the sofa where her mother is sitting – together they look at the photos)*
LAURA: Chien jaune. (Yellow dog.)
MOTHER: Chien jaune, oui. (Yes, yellow dog.)
LAURA: Chien jaune, les ph . . . et les . . . *(makes broken attempts to say words)* les pictures. *(pronounced 'pika')*
MOTHER: The picture.

There appears to be a relationship between Laura's mother's previous use of the English word 'pictures' in an utterance in which she mixes French and English, and Laura's later use of the same word in the mixed utterance, 'les picture' ('pika'). She even starts to attempt the French word 'photo' before switching to the English 'picture' – reasons underlying this case of mixing could well relate to less certain word knowledge for the French 'photo' than for the English 'picture', strengthened possibly by her mother's earlier use of English 'picture' in a mixed French/English utterance.

Children learning two languages simultaneously are seen by Genesee (1993) to use the same acquisition strategies used by monolingual learners, they develop differentiated language systems from the beginning and they are able to use language systems differentially in contextually sensitive ways. Juan-Garau and

Table 5.1 The developmental sequence of additional language acquisition in young children

Stage	Main features of communication and language use in the additional language
1	*Home language use* Some children may continue to use their home language in the additional language setting, such as at an English-speaking nursery.
2	*Nonverbal communication period* Once children are aware that their home language is not appropriate to all settings, they use nonverbal communication for purposes such as requesting objects and actions, getting attention, protesting and joking in the additional language settings. They start gathering information about the additional language and developing comprehension using strategies of observation and rehearsing.
3	*Early verbal period* Children start using the additional language in • telegraphic speech – combining a limited number of key words to make short phrases, such as Ahmed pencil/Ahmed blue pencil • formulaic speech – producing unanalysed chunks of the additional language in situations where they have heard others using them, for example 'tidy up time', 'dinner time' when appropriate.
4	*Productive language use* Once children have induced basic grammatical rules and acquired adequate vocabulary in the additional language, they can start constructing novel sentences and use the additional language creatively.

Source: Drury (2000).

extrovert children cracking the code of the additional language faster than those who are more withdrawn (Wong Fillmore 1979). Many professionals working with young sequential bilingual learners strongly believe that those involved in the education of these children need to know the stages expected in normal sequential bilingual acquisition, and need to be wary of a 'wait and see' approach towards bilingual children who remain quiet or appear to have significantly reduced verbal understanding over a reasonable period of time. Not taking action at the appropriate times by investigating the child's overall language profile (i.e. level of development in both languages) can result in some children remaining silent throughout their time at nursery. Watson and Cummins (1999) state that a six-month 'silent period' can be expected at the start of a child's time at nursery. Knowledge and awareness of issues concerning bilingual development can guard against its potential negative consequences (such as the loss of home language) and increase identification of difficulties in primary language development when they arise. Crutchley (1999) suggests that bilingual children have been under-represented as being in need of language learning support in the UK, due in part to inadequate identification of primary language difficulties as opposed to language differences.

The role of social interaction in sequential bilingual acquisition

The role of social interaction with peers and adults who speak the majority language is crucial in facilitating the bilingual child's acquisition of that language. Drury (2000) illustrates through a case study how a linguistic minority girl has a strong incentive to learn the new language of her nursery setting (English). She identifies the girl's use of active learning strategies, including practising and rehearsing language from the nursery setting, when playing at home. Use of these strategies is seen to help to consolidate the girl's learning. She is learning more than linguistic rules and new vocabulary, though. Through her observation of the nursery routines and rules, she learns new patterns of interaction with others, and internalizes what is expected of her and what is acceptable in this socio-cultural environment, thus reshaping her identity in the process (Drury 2000). The girl in Drury's case study is frequently socially isolated at nursery during the early stages of learning English, due to her inability to communicate with English-speaking peers in a way that they can respond to.

The girl's powerful motivation to learn the new language, which in turn will help her to make sense of the new setting and increase her participation in it, is observed in her play at home. She engages in role play, creating characters which engage in nursery-based activities, using language she has heard in the nursery setting. Her play thus reinforces the culture and the language of the nursery setting. The girl's English is far more creative and flexible in her play at home than when used in the nursery at this stage. As her confidence and competence in English grows, she starts to use *formulaic phrases* in play situations at nursery (for example 'No, mine') to protect her toys, but her utterances are largely ignored by peers at this stage.

This girl experiences the 'double bind' described by Tabor (Drury 2000) of being unable to interact successfully with peers due to limited language, and at the same time needing interaction opportunities in order to develop her language skills. She starts to interact successfully with adults, however, sharing conversations that are key to boosting her acquisition of English. In the light of these observations, Drury makes several suggestions for supporting bilingual language learners at nursery, which are outlined at the end of this chapter.

Each child is different, of course, and has a different profile of majority language learning, related (as noted above) to factors such as personality. Watson (1995) cites writers who have observed majority language learners who gain access to social interaction with peers at the early verbal period via formulaic social phrases such as 'My turn', 'Give it to me', which lead to further input of the additional language by peers, thus facilitating learning.

Cognitive academic language proficiency (CALP)

Once children have acquired basic interpersonal communicative skills in one language, they move on to what Cummins (1984) termed 'cognitive academic language proficiency' (CALP). CALP refers to a higher level of decontextualized language (used increasingly in the classroom as children move up the school),

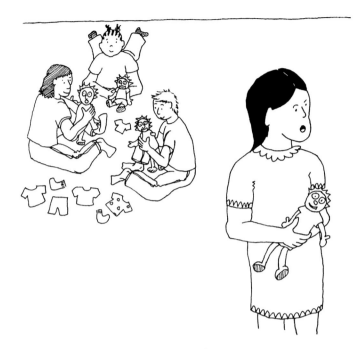

Figure 5.1 Young children at the early stages of learning an additional language may experience social isolation

development of literacy skills and a developing awareness about aspects of language in order to derive the meaning of a word, sentence or text. Cummins claims that children who have entered the CALP stage (this usually occurs between 4 and 5 years of age) and start acquiring an additional language at school, will take between one and two years to develop basic interpersonal communicative skill in that language. Children are thought to use their developing awareness about language generally to make sense of the additional language. It then takes between five and seven years to develop cognitive academic language proficiency in the additional language.

Language loss

Watson (1995) refers to the need for children to have attained a 'minimum threshold' in their (minority) home language before being able to benefit from instruction in an additional (majority) language. If their minority language is supported, children stand a better chance of moving into the CALP stage, which enables them to cope better with learning an additional language. This support also significantly reduces the risk of home language loss. This can arise when one language is abruptly replaced by another, without adequate continued input of the original language. This phenomenon has been termed '*subtractive bilingualism*' by

Lambert (1975). Subtractive bilingualism is strongly associated with negative consequences for cognition and language, particularly as children's progression in cognitive academic language proficiency is affected. Use of grammar and vocabulary in the minority language is negatively affected by loss of bilingual children's minority language. This loss is frequently seen to take place in the context of continued good verbal understanding, however, especially in conversation and informal situations (Anderson 1998).

Loss of children's minority language is widespread, despite the gradual rise in bilingualism. Malavé (1997) highlights the large number of children who lose their minority language shortly after they enter the English-speaking school environment. This is especially common in children whose families use both languages inter-changeably (Anderson 1998). Some such families shift their pattern of language use towards one resembling monolingualism once children start receiving instruction in English. If the minority language is not maintained at home to an adequate level, however, the risk of language loss is real.

Strategies used by sequential bilingual learners

Many strategies used by additional language learners are the same as those used by monolingual and simultaneous bilingual learners. Children are essentially active in trying out their hypotheses about language, overgeneralizing grammatical rules, and overextending and underextending word meanings. (For an explanation of these terms and examples of these strategies, see pages 56–60 and 109–111) Monolingual learners, like young additional language learners, also rehearse and practise new language in play. The girl in Drury's case study repeated and combined short phrases in English, extending them in the same way that monolingual learners do when making the transition between two-word utterances and three-word utterances in their expressive language development (see page 108), for example:

Little bit
Things back
Little bit back

Bilingualism and developmental language difficulties

Parents of bilingual children with developmental language learning difficulties (see Chapter 6 for a full account of these) often ask whether exposure to more than one language is advisable. Research has not yet proven that language acquisition by children with language learning difficulties is negatively affected by exposure to two languages (Watson 1995). However, Watson cites Carrow-Woolfolk and Lynch (1982) who recommend that children with severe difficulties should have exposure to only one language. These children's language-learning systems are considered to be inadequate for cracking the code of one language, let alone two. Children with less severe difficulties can be exposed to one language for the purposes of instruction, while their home language might differ. Duncan (1989), however, argues that disordered language learning systems need more and better language learning opportunities. Limiting these children's exposure to only one language (which is almost always the language of instruction and which may therefore differ from the language of the home) fails to meet the wider socio-cultural needs and realities of children from bilingual households.

Watson highlights several factors that impinge on decisions that parents make regarding raising their language-delayed child to be bilingual. These relate to parents' motivations and long-term vision of the language and cultural experiences they want to provide for their child. Parents who are committed to raising their language-delayed child to be bilingual are advised by Watson to provide them with exposure to both languages as early as possible. This is because simultaneous acquisition of two languages is generally less complex than sequential acquisition, and because sequential acquisition involves attainment of BICS and CALP taking longer. Parents who were able to provide dual language exposure early on to language-delayed children found that this helped their transition to school (Watson 1995). Of course, this option may not always be available to many parents. Services that provide therapeutic and educational support to language-delayed children and/or their parents in their home (minority) language might not be available, despite being highly desirable.

The level of parents' fluency in the two languages, which is related to feeling at ease in the language they speak and being able to maintain natural interactions with their child, is another important consideration. Watson describes fluency (language competence) as being able to hold conversations in formal and less formal settings, to talk about a range of topics including abstract ones, and to use language for reasoning (for example, explaining and problem-solving).

Watson advises that parents, when making decisions regarding language exposure to their language-delayed child, consider factors pertaining to their own fluency, commitment and motivation, and availability of services over and above the level of severity of their child's language difficulty. The potential benefits for children of being able to access two cultures are great, and Watson proposes that professionals support parents who opt to raise their language-delayed child bilingually.

Bilingualism, cognition and literacy development

Bilingualism and cognitive development

There have been highly controversial findings of studies looking at the links between bilingualism and cognitive development over the years (cited in Genesee 1993, Watson 1995, Malavé 1997). Studies conducted prior to the 1960s which reported negative effects of bilingualism, such as lower IQ, school achievement and language skills, were considered by later researchers to have been undertaken in subtractive bilingual environments in which students had not developed an adequate level of linguistic competence in their home language before receiving academic instruction in the additional, majority language. This factor was not taken into consideration when interpreting findings.

Later studies revealed that many bilingual learners with high levels of linguistic proficiency in both languages had better concept formation, social skills, creativity, logical reasoning, *categorization* skills, cognitive flexibility and metalinguistic awareness. Cummins (1981, cited in Genesee 1993) proposed that these types of differences in cognitive performance are not observed in bilinguals who have lower levels of linguistic proficiency.

Against this research background, Bialystok and Herman make the following plea:

> It would be surprising indeed if bilingualism conferred an influence so broad in scope and so global in mechanism that it stood in some simple relation to a complex process such as cognitive development. These relationships must be examined at a more finely tuned level of analysis: what is it about bilingualism that has what effects on which aspects of cognitive growth? The formulation of the question that compels us to choose between two broad and opposite options, namely, that bilingualism either helps or hinders cognitive growth, is not helpful.
>
> (Bialystok and Herman 1999: 35)

The multidimensional nature of bilingualism should preclude it from being viewed and used as an independent variable in research, and as such cannot be used in research to test out differences or similarities between groups of monolingual speakers and groups of bilingual speakers. Fine-tuning the level of analysis includes taking into account factors such as languages spoken, relative levels of proficiency, patterns of language use and socio-cultural expectations. For example, play is frequently used as a means of considering aspects of cognitive development in children by clinicians, educators and researchers; it is essential that culturally appropriate play materials (for example articles of cutlery, food and clothing) are presented to children in these circumstances, in the interests of validity.

With improvements in research methodology and greater attention paid towards the multidimensional nature of 'bilingualism', studies looking at links between cognitive development in bilingual speakers point towards overall greater cognitive flexibility and awareness of language (Hakuta 1990) than in monolingual speakers. At the age of 2 years and 9 months, Laura was frequently asked by her mother to reflect on the languages she was in the process of learning. This is illustrated in the following conversation, held mostly in French (English translations are in brackets):

LAURA: Sable. (Sand.)
MOTHER: Yes . . . Comment c'est en grec? (How do you say that in Greek?)
LAURA: Uh? Uh? Uh? (What? What? What?)
MOTHER: Comment c'est en grec? (How do you say that in Greek?)
LAURA: I don't know.

MOTHER: Yes you do . . . sable? (Sand?)
LAURA: Simi. (Cloud.)
MOTHER: Non (No) . . . simi (cloud) – ça c'est le nuage (that's cloud) . . . come on . . . et en grec? (and in Greek?)

The need that bilingual learners have for separating out the *form* of language from the meaning, in order to separate out the two language systems being learned, is thought to contribute to their enhanced metalinguistic development (Hakuta 1990).

Bilingualism and literacy development

A question frequently asked by researchers concerns the relationship between bilingualism and the development of literacy skills – is bilingualism a factor in learning to read? Bearing in mind the need to fine tune the level of analysis, Bialystok and Herman have started to formulate a response to this question supported by the results of studies in which they separated out factors such as the type of experiences individuals have had in which languages, the levels of proficiency in each language, the relationship between the languages (French and Spanish are far closer than French and Japanese) and the type of writing system in each language (Bialystok and Herman 1999). In consideration of these factors, Bialystok and Herman looked at the social, cognitive and linguistic dimensions of emergent literacy skills (see pages 145–146 for further information on these) in different groups of bilingual children.

The social dimension

Previous experience with books, through being read stories in particular, has a positive effect on children's ability to develop narrative skills which include the use of a decontextualized, literate language style, logical organization of text and cohesive devices such as use of pronouns. For bilingual children, this effect is language-specific – that is, they develop these skills in the language in which they have had book sharing experiences. Although greater flexibility has been observed in other aspects of bilingual children's language development, they were not seen to generalize a literate style of language from one language to another if they had not had previous experience of book and story sharing in that language. This finding has important implications for encouraging storytelling and book sharing in each of a bilingual child's languages in order to support the move towards true cognitive academic language proficiency that requires a minimum threshold of competence in each language.

The cognitive dimension

Bilingual children's concepts of print, or their understanding of the purpose of squiggles on a page, and whether there is any difference between the development of their and monolingual children's concept of print, is another subject of interest. Bialystok and Herman (1999) report studies that suggest bilingual learners pay greater attention to the relationship between the form of a word (how it is written or spoken) and its meaning. This awareness enables them to see a one-to-one relationship between the printed form of a word and its pictorial referent more reliably than monolingual children at an early age. Bilingual children learning two different writing systems (French and Chinese, or English and Japanese, for example) develop a better understanding of the function of print (be it letters or characters) at an earlier age than both monolingual speakers and bilingual children learning only one writing system (French and English, for example). This advantage, demonstrated in 5-year-old Chinese/English bilingual children who could successfully connect the number of sounds in a word with the number of letters needed to write it, is thought to be related to the experience of needing to learn the principles of two completely different writing systems (Bialystok and Herman 1999).

The linguistic dimension

Phonological awareness, or the conscious awareness of the sounds of a language, is widely acknowledged as supporting children's early literacy development. Once again, the question of whether bilingual children demonstrate a significant difference in these skills against those who are monolingual has been the subject of much research. Once again, factors such as the relation between the two languages and the type of task involved determined results. Even limited exposure to another language at an early age yielded a slight advantage over monolingual children in tasks requiring sensitivity to sound properties of words – this effect was neutralized by the time children were 6, however. Bialystok and Herman suggest this may be due to instruction in phonological awareness delivered to all children in the first year at school. These and other results suggest some early advantage to bilinguals, when the sound systems of the two languages resemble each other (French and Spanish, or Italian and English, for example). This effect is not generalized with reliability to bilingual children whose languages have a significant disparity in their sound systems, such as French and Chinese.

Environmental factors impacting on bilingual acquisition

Quality and quantity of language input

It is now widely recognized that consistent and adequate input in both languages is necessary for both simultaneous and sequential learners in order to achieve balanced bilingualism. Discussion of the risks associated with reduced input in one language can be found on pages 166–167.

Social and cultural factors

Schools are widely recognized as reflecting the cultural values and expectations of middle classes more than any other group in society. Middle and upper class linguistic minority immigrants find it easier to adapt to the majority culture's educational systems, while all lower socio-economic groups find it harder to identify with the educational culture of the school (Madhani 1994). Students belonging to those groups that feel most disenfranchised from the educational system, such as the poorest immigrant and refugee groups, show highest levels of school under-achievement. This continues to be the case despite positive changes in the levels of provision for the needs of bilingual children in schools and attitudes towards bilingualism in many educational establishments in the UK (Crutchley 1999).

While there are moves in many areas of the UK, for example, away from a limited frame of educational reference reflecting white middle class cultural values, towards a multicultural and multilingual one that is intended to increase access for all children (Crutchley 1999), this entails a fundamental and long-term shift in curriculum content and attitudes and as such will take a long time to achieve; meanwhile the situation for these children remains complex. In an attempt to illustrate this complexity, Crutchley cites writers who variously specify the challenging complication of starting to learn the language of instruction at the same time that the instruction commences; a possible mismatch between home and school cultural expectations and patterns of language use; overt, covert and institutional racism and adverse social and economic circumstances.

There is agreement in the literature that the quality of the relationship between the bilingual child and the adult speaker of the additional language is highly influential in the child's acquisition of that language. Krashen (1981) proposed that a number of 'affective variables' serve to facilitate additional language acquisition. These include motivation, self-confidence, a low level of anxiety and a good self-image. Deficiencies in these areas can negatively impact additional language acquisition by forming a 'mental block' that prevents language input, even highly comprehensible input, from being used for purposes of acquisition. Positive affect is more likely to exist when the majority language speaking adult is sensitive to the needs of the bilingual learner, encouraging requests for clarification when speakers misunderstand each other, and adapting what is said to suit each other's level of understanding.

There are, of course, many other relevant factors impacting on affective variables, including the fundamental question of identity. Madhani (1994: 12) cites Halliday's (1975) claim that culture is carried through language, and cultural identity is developed and reinforced through using language. In the light of this, she asks, 'What is the effect on linguistic minority children's cultural identity when they enter the school environment and are surrounded by another language and another culture? The effect can only be profound.' Baker (1996: 48) refers to studies in the UK which suggested that immigrants ask of themselves 'whether they are Asian or British, or incipient Europeans, or have no or little identity, or whether they are a mix of the host and the native culture.' Such lack of clarity around this issue of identity extends to children, who may experience conflicts of loyalties as they acquire the values, attitudes and behaviours of the majority culture in the course of learning its language (Baker 1996). Some bilingual immigrants in predominantly monolingual western countries are reported to experience divided loyalties, a sense of rootlessness, shame and guilt in connection with their bilingual status (Baker 1996). Watson (1995) cites Cummins' claim that parents' ambivalence towards the majority culture or shame towards the minority culture can impact negatively on their children's language development.

Implications for supporting bilingual acquisition in young children

In order to prevent against language loss, promote the transition from basic inter-personal communicative skills to cognitive academic linguistic proficiency in both languages and build self-confidence as a bilingual speaker, bilingual children benefit from specific types of support. The following suggestions, which draw on work by Watson and Cummins (1999), Rettig (1995) and Drury (2000), are proposed:

- Parents should be strongly encouraged to continue providing input in the minority home language through talking, playing, singing and especially storytelling and book sharing activities.
- A positive attitude towards families' bilingual status and towards the languages they speak should be fostered and communicated to children and parents.
- Majority language speaking educators need to provide additional language learners with opportunities for one-to-one interaction with adults to help their acquisition of the majority language.
- Majority language speaking educators can facilitate additional language learning by using short phrases, gestures and other visual cues to support the linguistic signal.
- Majority language speaking educators should engage additional language learners in teacher-led small group work involving a high level of contextual support for children's developing comprehension.
- Children are helped to internalize language through music and songs, which is a non-threatening way for additional language learners to learn the majority language.
- Bilingual assistant and support staff should be used in education to help young additional language learners understand what is socially and culturally expected of them, to support their language development and to provide continuity between the home and educational environments.
- Social interaction with majority language speaking peers in education settings should be facilitated through strategies such as teaching early social phrases, pairing minority and majority speaking children off together and supporting play in small groups of children.
- Consistency and predictability should be provided regarding the rules and

routines of the educational setting, thus helping minority language learners adjust to it.

•   Account should be taken in the educational setting of all children's home environments and cultural backgrounds through including multicultural activities and materials as part of the daily classroom experience. In particular, use should be made of dramatic play, cooking and music (see Rettig 1995 for a detailed account of these).

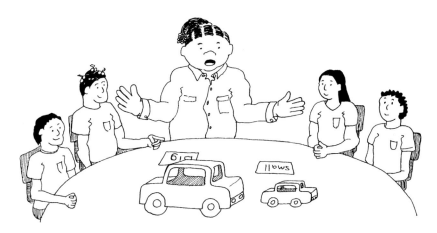

Figure 5.2 Nursery teacher leading a language group with bilingual children

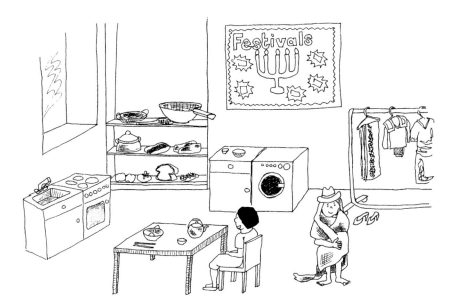

Figure 5.3 Nursery classroom reflecting multicultural experiences and backgrounds

Summary of Chapter 5

Bilingualism

1   Several definitions of bilingualism have been proposed – a useful one is Madhani's (1994), 'understanding and using two or more languages to varying degrees at various times'.

2   It is the norm to learn and use more than one language in most countries of the world – bilingualism is, however, regarded as exceptional by many monolingual inhabitants of the UK, USA and Australasia.

3   There are identifiable patterns of language use which relate to interaction variables among families who raise simultaneously bilingual children from birth.

4   There are identifiable patterns of language use which relate closely to the purpose and location of the interaction in linguistic minority communities, regardless of the languages involved.

5   Proficiency in a certain language is closely related to the individual's use of that language; some speakers maintain productive use of more than one language while others might understand more than one language yet only use one productively.

6   There is evidence of increasing bilingualism in western countries, due primarily to large-scale international migration. However, loss of minority languages can occur in a linguistic minority community within two or three generations of immigration.

Features of bilingual speech and the patterns and stages of bilingual acquisition

7   Children may learn two languages from birth (simultaneous bilingualism) or may learn an additional language (usually that spoken by the majority culture in the country in which they live) once basic interpersonal communicative skill has been achieved in their home language (sequential bilingualism).

8   Bilingual adults mix words, intonation patterns, pronunciation and grammar from their two languages both within sentences and over a conversation. Code mixing and code switching are seen as sophisticated language behaviours in mature bilingual speakers.

9   Mature bilingual speakers often speak one language with greater proficiency than another; how a speaker expresses himself in his weaker language might be influenced by specific factors from the dominant language.

10   Children learning two languages from birth approach the task with no fundamental difference in their cognitive abilities, knowledge of the world, social understanding or communicative competence from monolingual children of the same age.

11 Some researchers believe simultaneous bilingual learners develop two differentiated language systems from birth, while others believe that two differentiated systems develop out of an original unitary language system.

12 The amount of code mixing and switching in adult speech is thought to influence occurrence of mixing in young bilingual learners.

13 Parental support of a child's weaker, or minority, language is thought to be closely linked to the level of productivity in that language by the child.

14 Sequential bilingual learners use what they have learned about language and communication to help them start learning an additional language.

15 There is a developmental sequence to additional language learning in young children, with varying levels of nonverbal and verbal communication.

16 Young sequential bilingual learners are often in the position of being unable to interact successfully with majority language speaking peers due to limited language, and at the same time need interaction opportunities in order to develop their language skills.

17 Sequential language learners need to have developed a minimum threshold of basic interpersonal communicative competence in one language before they can successfully receive instruction in another language.

18 An adequate and consistent level of input in a sequential bilingual learner's two languages is necessary to enable them to progress in both languages to a level of cognitive academic language proficiency, necessary for learning in school in later years.

Bilingualism, cognition and literacy development

19 There is thought to be generally greater levels of cognitive flexibility and awareness about language in bilinguals than monolinguals.

20 Any relationships that exist between bilingualism and the development of literacy are dependent on which languages are involved, which writing systems, which sound systems, the type of experiences individuals have had in each language and levels of proficiency in each language. As with the relationship between bilingualism and cognitive development, it is not possible to treat bilingualism as an independent variable.

Environmental factors impacting on bilingual acquisition

21 Sequential bilingual learners are often faced with multiple challenges in predominantly monolingual, western countries relating to their cultural and linguistic identity; cognitive, cultural and linguistic demands made of them upon entering the school system; and racism and economic factors.

22 A trusting and positive relationship with adult majority language speakers is necessary for acquisition of the majority language to take place, but is not sufficient on its own.

23 Professionals involved in working with young bilingual learners need to know how to support their developing language systems, to be aware of the potential and long-term negative consequences of subtractive bilingualism and to acknowledge that these children have additional needs to monolingual learners.

Problems developing speech, language and communication

6

- ○ The nature of childhood communication difficulties and ways of describing them.
- ○ Types of speech, language and communication skills that children might develop.
- ○ Understanding childhood communication difficulties in terms of environmental and internal factors.
- ○ Summary of key points.

The nature of communication difficulties

The multi-factorial nature of communication difficulties

It needs to be stressed that childhood communication difficulties are usually the result of a number of contributory factors impinging on the child's development. This is partly due to the multi-factorial nature of human communication (see the Introduction to this book, pages 1–22) and partly due to the interaction of contributory factors within and external to the child, some of which might be instrumental in exacerbating or maintaining a difficulty. Thus a hearing child of deaf parents who experiences plenty of normal human communication through interaction with her parents yet hears less clear spoken language in their presence might well develop normal speech and language (Mogford and Bishop 1993b). Such a child would usually be exposed to spoken language from other sources, too. A child in similar circumstances, but who is also chronically neglected by her parents and who therefore does not experience normal human communication through interaction with her parents, is at risk for developing speech and language difficulties. It is necessary to treat each child as unique with respect to the likelihood of different factors impacting on the development of their speech, language and communication and not to make judgments on how a particular child's speech or language might develop based solely on previous experience of children who share the same diagnosis, for example *hearing impairment*. Mogford and Bishop (1993b) additionally point to the need to consider how constitutional differences between children impact on their communication skills development when faced with potentially adverse internal or environmental factors.

Describing childhood communication difficulties

Primary, associated and acquired communication difficulties

Communication difficulties might arise in association with other conditions which affect wider areas of development, such as *autism*, *learning difficulties* and *cerebral palsy*. Some communication difficulties arise in the absence of other areas of developmental difficulty and are due to primary problems with speech and language processing. Children with these difficulties fail to develop speech or language normally for no apparent reason, i.e. their difficulty cannot be explained by *environmental deprivation*, *sensory impairments*, learning difficulties, or physical or psychiatric problems (Mogford and Bishop 1993b). Other children may acquire communication difficulties at some point in childhood, for example as a result of brain damage due to *head injury* or some other cause (Lees and Unwin 1991).

Delay, disorder or difference?

When there is a difference affecting the rate or manner of a child's communication skills development relative to that of other children of the same age, that difference might be described as a *delay* or a *disorder*. Delayed development refers to communication skills which are developing in the same way, but at a slower pace than in other children of the same age. Delay might or might not also be apparent in other areas of the child's development, such as their motor, cognitive or social skills. A disorder of speech, language or communication development implies a difference in the course or pattern of development to that normally expected and observed in most other children of the same age, i.e. as distinct from the development occurring in essentially the same way, but at a slower rate. Some writers (for example Paul 1995) prefer to use the term 'disorder' to refer to all childhood communication difficulties. Paul considers the term 'delayed' to be overly simplistic as it does not take into account the difference in experiences and development that a child with 'delayed' communication skills will have undergone relative to their peers. Regardless of whether a child develops communication at a slower pace and/or in a different way from most other children the same age, the child can be said to have a difficulty developing their communication skills.

Environmental and internal factors contributing to communication difficulties

The range of developmental and acquired conditions that might impact on a child's developing communication skills is extensive and beyond the scope of this book to describe. It is possible, however, to revisit the environmental and internal factors which contribute to the development of children's communication skills (these were introduced in the Introduction, pages 17–18, and are schematized in Figure 6.1) and to illustrate how disturbances in these might impact on speech, language or communication development.

Once again, it is important to stress the multi-factorial nature of communication difficulties; the following section is subdivided into headings that should not give the misleading impression that communication difficulties can be traced to a single major cause, or require a single approach in intervention. It is necessary to consider how different environmental and internal factors might impact on a child's whole speech, language and communication system but equally, if not more important to remember that 'perhaps these [communication] disorders arise when a specific combination of adverse factors co-occur in a single child. Factors which on their own have no impact on language development might assume significance in combination' (Mogford and Bishop 1993b: 260).

Environmental factors

In the context of normal human communication

The question that needs to be asked is, 'Can a child's speech, language or communication be negatively affected due to environmental factors?' When considering communication, environmental factors need to be defined in terms of the communication, language and speech input that children are exposed to over the course of their development. Deprivation of general experiences, however, can lead to reduced learning, concept development and knowledge about the world, resulting in restricted language development.

Findings from several writers who have variously approached the question of environmental impact on communication development are summarized in Mogford and Bishop (1993b), who report that children's development in these areas is remarkably robust in the face of apparently adverse environmental conditions. These conditions relate to a reduction in the amount of spoken language the children are exposed to relative to other children the same age. For example, hearing children of deaf parents whose first language is sign have less exposure to spoken language than other children of the same age. Bilingual children have no less exposure to spoken language per se, but have less exposure to each of the languages they are learning than monolingual children of the same age. Twins sometimes present with mild language delay, which is considered to be related to a reduction in personalized episodes of interaction that are central to the establishment of joint attention and

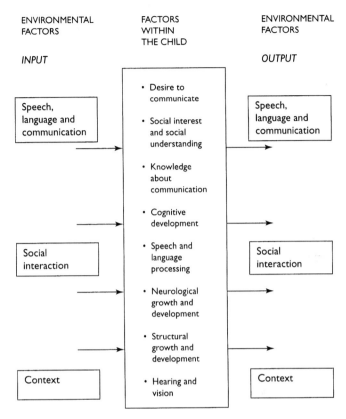

Figure 6.1 Internal and environmental factors contributing to speech, language and communication development in children

maintenance of conversations between children and caregivers (study cited by Mogford 1993). This is because caregivers have finite resources and are physically unable to respond consistently in a way that acknowledges each twin's focus of attention. However, none of these conditions has resulted in a greater likelihood of speech, language or communication difficulty in the longer term, everything else being equal. 'Everything else' roughly translates into normal human communication (reciprocal social interaction, adequate opportunities for interaction, positive emotional relationship with carers).

Postnatal depression

Research findings indicate both immediate and long-term impacts on various areas of development (including communication skills) in children of women who experience depression within the first few months of the baby's life (Murray 2001). Emotional unresponsiveness in mothers, due to *postnatal depression* during these first few months, carries a high risk of later *emotional regulation* and *attachment* difficulties and poorer performance on developmental tests in children. Depressed mothers vocalize less, respond more slowly, use more variable utterances and pauses and are less likely to use an exaggerated range of pitch characteristic of speech directed to infants (variously termed 'motherese' and 'child directed talk'; see the Introduction, pages 19–21 for further discussion). Studies of mother–infant face-to-face interactions with depressed mothers also show that they are less sensitively attuned to their babies than mothers who are not depressed (Murray 2001). Depressed mothers were found to be overly remote or intrusive during interactions with their babies (Murray 1992). Either of these interaction styles can impact on the child's development. Mothers whose speech focuses on the baby's experience at 2 months, rather than directing the baby to do what she wants, results in the baby achieving a better score on cognitive tasks at 9 months (Murray 2001). This effect echoes finding by Tomasello and Todd (1983) (see this volume, pages 50–51), whereby adult attempts to direct a child's attention or behaviour were found to be negatively correlated with the proportion of names for objects in a child's vocabulary at 21 months, and that when mothers name objects that are already within a child's focus of attention, the child has a greater proportion of object names in their vocabulary at 21 months.

This effect continues through to the school years; mothers who had greater difficulty seeing things from the baby's perspective had children who were at a greater risk of cognitive delay at the age of 5 (Murray 2001). Cognitive delays in children are usually associated with speech and language delays. Murray (1992) also found a higher rate of behaviour difficulties (sleep problems, temper tantrums, eating and separation problems) in 18-month-old children whose mothers had been depressed. In the face of these and related findings, Murray stresses that there are depressed mothers who have good relationships with their babies, and non-depressed mothers who have poor relationships with their babies. The presence of postnatal depression, however (especially in the context of deprived circumstances), increases the risk of a negative impact on children's development (Murray 2001). For a wider discussion on the impact of postnatal depression on child development, including the development of communication skills, see Murray and Andrews (2000).

Abuse and neglect

When normal human communication breaks down or is absent, as in the cases of abusive and abnormal relationships between children and their caregivers, the development of communication skills becomes vulnerable. Children who are or have been *physically*, *emotionally* or *sexually abused*, or who have been *neglected* are at risk of having problems developing speech, language and communication skills (Law and Conway 1990), especially relating to how they use their language and their desire to communicate.

Except in cases where abuse has a direct impact on the child (as in damage to the voice box due to strangulation, for example), neglect is found to have a more pervasive and powerful effect on language development. This is especially so where the relationship between parent and child is seriously abnormal and interaction has effectively broken down. Fox *et al.* (1988) found a direct association between neglect and language difficulties, including verbal comprehension. The chronic nature of neglect on the children studied was thought to play a significant role in their difficulties acquiring language. Egeland *et al.* (1983) discovered that different types of maltreatment suffered by babies from their parents resulted in different patterns of presenting behaviours at follow-up four years later. Physically abused children had higher levels of distractibility, lower persistence and lower enthusiasm for teaching tasks. Neglected children had low self-esteem, were the most unhappy and had difficulties organizing themselves when approaching and completing tasks.

Case study 6.1 Belal

Belal was 4½ when his mother brought him for an assessment of his communication skills. He came from a minority language speaking family and was growing up bilingual. His mother was a housewife and his father worked in a restaurant. He was previously known to the service and had been discharged (due to non-attendance) and re-referred twice by his teacher due to persisting concerns about his attention and language development that were affecting his learning. During assessment, which was conducted in both languages, the most salient feature of his behaviour was his high level of distractibility, poor listening and inability to attend visually to tasks. His skills in both languages were significantly delayed for his age. He achieved a lower score in one language assessment than he had nine months previously, raising serious questions about the possibility of a degenerative condition. He was not observed to initiate any interaction with his mother or the examiner. Shortly after that meeting it was revealed that Belal had been subjected to repeated bouts of physical abuse at the hands of his father.

There is no intention of drawing a link between bilingual families or ethnic minorities and increased likelihood of abuse or neglect. Rather, Belal's case was selected in an attempt to illustrate the complex picture that emerges when considering the various influences on an individual child's development.

When considering the impact of abuse or neglect on the child's communication skills development, it is necessary to consider other factors that may also have a causal role. As a group, children with developmental difficulties are more vulnerable to maltreatment than other children – those with communication difficulties can present as unrewarding and frustrating interaction partners; some have *oromotor* dysfunction with resultant feeding (and speech) problems which may have a dramatic impact on the parent–child relationship (Mathieson *et al.* 1989). It is also necessary, then, to consider how the child's behaviour and communication impacts on their environment and whether a pre-existing communication difficulty is exacerbated because of a high number of negative interactions with caregivers.

Law and Conway (1990) acknowledge the extreme difficulty associated with attempting to attribute a communication difficulty to abuse or neglect, due to the great variation within normal language development among children and the multi-factorial nature of communication and childhood communication difficulties. They advise professionals who are required to offer expert evidence to substantiate their opinions regarding the role of abuse or neglect in speech and language behaviour:

- to look for arrested language development (frequently co-occurring with other areas of arrested development, such as growth)
- to consider if there have been significant changes in the way a child uses language, such as an increase in sexualized language
- to consider if the child uses language as a defence against the world and to prevent close contact.

Encouragingly, many children who have been abused or neglected show improvements in speech and language development when placed in a more normal environment (Law and Conway 1990, Mogford and Bishop 1993b). Law and Conway recommend that these children's communication skills be regularly reviewed throughout their care arrangements, as results of assessments can contribute towards gauging the level of success of a child's placement.

To conclude this section, it is necessary to clarify that it is only in the cases of extreme abuse and neglect that the development of children's communication skills is at risk. The majority of parents whose children have problems communicating have not done, or omitted to do, anything that has caused their child's difficulty. It is very important to convey this to parents.

Internal factors

Desire to communicate

Some children do not communicate verbally in certain contexts, especially those where there is an expectation to speak (school, for example), despite using speech at home.

Several reasons might underlie and perpetuate this behaviour, relating to environmental and internal factors (Johnson and Wintgens 2001). There is usually anxiety associated with speaking, sometimes associated speech and language difficulties; there may be a family history of anxiety or of speech and language difficulty and there may be negative models of communication within the family (Cline and Baldwin 1994, Imich 1998, Johnson and Wintgens 2001). The group of children described in this section are termed '*selectively mute*' in the 1994 edition of the *Diagnostic and Statistical Manual of Mental Disorders* (DSM-IV) (American Psychiatric Association 1994), implying that they do not speak in 'select' situations (Johnson and Wintgens 2001).

Selective mutism is more common in girls, especially from ethnic or linguistic minority families and in families who are geographically or socially isolated (Cline and Baldwin 1994). Onset is often insidious and occurs around the time that children are expected to speak more with a wider range of people outside of the home, and at a time when most children of the same age have developed fluent conversational speech – between the ages of 3 and 5.

Identification of children who are selectively mute is important as it gets harder to treat the longer it is left, and treatment in younger children often has positive results (Johnson and Wintgens 2001). Untreated and persistent selective mutism, or an apparently milder reluctance to communicate, can have serious and long lasting effects, such as feelings of inadequacy and vulnerability which Johnson and Wintgens (2001) state are hard to shake off in later life. Reluctant communicators include those who are not mute in specific contexts yet who respond minimally in them (and usually initiate verbal interaction infrequently, if at all), and are vulnerable to being overlooked (Johnson and Wintgens 2001). They are at risk of developing mutism and other anxiety-related behaviours over several years (see Case study 6.2). Johnson and Wintgens (2001), who note that onset of selective mutism is often associated with starting at school or nursery, advise that two or three months after a child has started and had the opportunity to settle in and yet is not speaking should be the time for an initial meeting between parents and relevant professionals.

Case study 6.2 Rebecca

Rebecca, who had severe speech and language difficulty, started at nursery at the age of 4. She had always been a good communicator who spoke freely at home, and her family had got used to the way she spoke. However, after starting nursery it gradually became clear that she was reluctant to communicate freely with adults outside the home. This reluctance did not go away, and by the age of 8 she had developed some inappropriate ways of interacting with adults, such as turning her whole body away, throwing things to gain their attention, and not returning greetings or offering thanks when necessary. She had no difficulty in communicating and speaking with other children she was familiar with. Treatment of Rebecca's speech and language disorder was successful in many ways, but the emotional and psychological aspects had been largely overlooked.

Children who are selectively mute are not the only ones who have a reduced desire to communicate, of course. It is important to differentiate between those children who use speech only in a circumscribed set of contexts, and those children who do not use speech across contexts due to another developmental or psychiatric disorder. Any child who appears to genuinely not want to engage in communication (verbal or nonverbal) with others needs careful handling; the problem should be discussed with parents and the expertise of relevant professionals should be sought if necessary.

Knowledge about social behaviour and communication

Children who have disturbances in their ability to relate to other people will experience difficulties in understanding and responding appropriately to communication and in using language effectively, especially for social purposes. Hence the dual grouping of these internal factors in this section. Of course, there is potential interaction among all internal and environmental factors, but knowledge about social interaction and knowledge about communication are inextricably linked (Happé 1994). Knowledge about communication refers to the various purposes one uses communication for (see Table 2.2, page 64, and Table 4.1, page 136, for reasons why young children communicate), and to knowing how to respond to other people's communication. Social understanding is about knowing what motivates people's behaviour on emotional and social levels. The ability to represent or imagine states of mind in ourselves and other people helps us to make sense of situations (especially social situations) and of other people's behaviour. 'Mental states' refer to an individual's intentions, feelings, beliefs, desires and plans. Understanding other people in terms of their mental states is central to the process of human communication. This ability, which has been termed 'mind-reading' (Happé 1994, Baron-Cohen 1999), is fundamental to relating to other people. Mind-reading enables us to think about a situation from another person's perspective or point of view (Happé 1994). An effect of an inability to mind-read is illustrated in Example 6.1.

Example 6.1 Illustration of an inability to mind-read

A teacher is in the classroom with two 5-year-old boys, Adam and Neil. Neil is autistic. The teacher shows the boys a ball which she then places in a box on the table, replacing the lid on the box. There is also a basket on the table with nothing in it. Both containers are opaque. She asks Adam to leave the room for a little while. When Adam is out of the room, she removes the ball from the box, replaces the lid and places it in the basket. She asks Neil, 'Where will Adam look for the ball?' Neil replies, 'In the basket'. He lacks the ability to mind-read, or 'get inside the head' of the other boy, whose state of knowledge about the ball is different to his own, which is the 'real' one.

Research by Baron-Cohen *et al.* (1985) concluded that, as a group, children with autism have a unique deficit in their social understanding: they do not understand that other people have mental states which can be different from the state of the real world and different from their own mental state.

Baron-Cohen *et al.* (1985) found ability to mind-read in normally developing 4-year-olds and children with *Down's syndrome* of similar mental abilities. This finding has been replicated in a number of subsequent and related studies. The triad of impairments that lies at the core of autism – problems with social interaction, with social communication and with social imagination (which includes difficulties with flexible thinking and imaginative play) (Wing and Gould 1979) – is considered by Frith *et al.* (1991) and Happé (1994) to be largely due to an inability to mind-read. Impaired imaginative play, for example, is thought to be related to an inability to represent mentally the components of imaginative play – the actions, thoughts, beliefs and behaviours of self and others. It follows that if these are not represented mentally they cannot be transferred into a child's play, drawings or language. The social impairment results from a lack of understanding that people are separate beings with independent minds. The communication disorders of autism result from an impaired ability to conceptualize intentions and make the connection between what other people say and do, and what they think (Happé 1994).

All children with autism demonstrate this 'triad of impairments' (Wing and Gould 1979) but differ in terms of the severity of the disorder. Some autistic children do not develop speech and some develop sophisticated language skills. Although many autistic individuals are able to formulate long sentences and use a wide vocabulary, the way they use language is qualitatively different from how other people use language. This difference is largely down to reduced social awareness and a reduced appreciation of what communication is for, over and above meeting one's needs through regulating other people's behaviour.

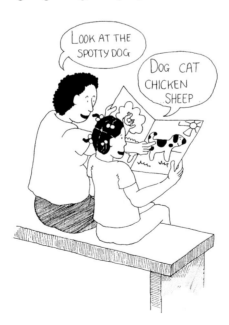

Figure 6.2 For some children, conversations with other people are hard, even though they have learned how to talk

So far, research has not identified children whose primary difficulty is in understanding and using communication appropriately, but whose social and imaginative development are unaffected (Happé 1994). There are, however, children who have specific difficulty developing language and who might also have problems with social interaction and using communication effectively and appropriately. It is necessary to consider all aspects of a child's speech, language and communication when problems in one area are suspected.

Problems in social and communication development might be described as a 'social communication disorder'. Some children who are not autistic have social communication disorders. Unusual or bizarre ways of relating to people, of responding to communication, of using communication and of using language are indicators of a social communication disorder. It is important to remember that the more subtle and apparently 'mild' social and communication impairments are frequently overlooked and misunderstood (see page 204 for a description of Daniel; see also Lees and Urwin 1991: 72).

Although the focus of this section has been on primary deficits in social interaction and communication, it is important to point out that problems with socializing and communication arise in association with a range of conditions including speech and language processing problems, attention disorders, and also in association with inappropriate environmental input.

Cognitive development

Cognitive development is to do with the acquisition and retention of knowledge about the world through the process of learning. Learning involves processes such as attention, perception, memory, problem-solving and thinking in general (Gross 1992). Children with cognitive impairment, or 'learning difficulties', take longer to learn and have less efficient ways of learning than other children of the same age. Children with learning difficulties develop more slowly in all areas of their development than their peers, arriving at each stage of their development at a later age and staying there for longer.

Children differ in terms of the severity of their cognitive impairment. No direct link between cognition and language has yet been made (Rondal 1993), but slowness in children's conceptual development and other areas of cognition is associated with delays in developing communication, language and speech. There is some evidence that cognitive and linguistic development generally progress parallel to each other. However, the development of some children's cognition and language appears to be unconnected to each other (Bernstein Ratner 1989). Each child has a different learning profile to another, but there are also specific learning profiles to some developmental learning difficulties, such as Down's syndrome (Buckley 2000), with characteristic strengths and weaknesses. Many children with learning difficulties follow an essentially normal, but delayed pattern of development in their communicative abilities, with later onset, lower final level of achievement but similar stages of acquisition (Bernstein Ratner 1989).

Children with learning difficulties take longer to make links between things in the world and the words that represent them, hence their language development is slower than other children's. There is some evidence to suggest that children with learning difficulties experience more difficulty learning to use grammar and less difficulty learning how to use language for communicative purposes, and that their verbal understanding might exceed predictions made from their cognitive level of ability (Bernstein Ratner 1989). Many also have hearing and speech difficulties.

There are many different causes of learning difficulties, and most children who have problems with general learning also have problems developing speech and language. Identification of children with delayed speech, language and communication development associated with learning difficulties sometimes occurs due to concerns raised about other areas of development, such as delayed attainment of motor milestones, and sometimes these are the main area of concern initially. In other cases it is obvious from birth that a child has a learning difficulty, as in children with Down's syndrome.

Children who are known to have learning difficulties will require a full assessment of their communication skills in order that appropriate advice and intervention can be offered. Some children who have learning difficulties also have unusual patterns of development in their communication, language and speech, constituting a disorder. This needs to be borne in mind as a different approach to meeting these children's needs might be necessary.

Children's play skills progress in association with their cognitive development and can therefore provide a good indication of some cognitive skills (symbolic development and concept development, for example). This can be especially useful when working with nonverbal children, or with reluctant speakers with whom it might be hard to establish verbal interaction.

Cognitive impairment can arise during childhood for a number of reasons, including accident (for example a head injury) and disease (for example some degenerative diseases), and might be generalized to affect all learning or have more specific effects.

Speech and language processing

Problems in speech and language processing can arise in association with cognitive impairment, conditions which involve primary impairments in the development of social and communication skills (such as autism) and other types of neuro-developmental problems (i.e. arising from problems in development of the brain, such as *childhood epilepsy*) (Lees *et al.* 1991). Dysfluent speech (stammering) is thought to arise due to an interaction between problems with planning and processing speech and language, and other factors such as too high demands being made of children and high parental expectations for good speech or behaviour (Starkweather 1987). Some children, however, have specific difficulty developing language and/or speech and what may originally look like a delay in a child's speech and language skills emerges as a *language disorder*. Lees *et al.* (1991) provide the following definition of this type of difficulty, which is sometimes called '*specific language impairment*':

> A language disorder is that language profile which, although it may be associated with a history of hearing, learning, environmental and emotional difficulties, cannot be attributed to any one of these alone, or even just the sum of these effects, and in which one or more of the following is also seen:
>
> 1 A close positive family history of specific difficulty in language development.
> 2 Evidence of cerebral dysfunction, either during development or by the presence of neurological signs.
> 3 A mismatch between the various subsystems of language in relation to other aspects of cognitive development.
> 4 A failure to catch up these differences with 'generalized' language help.
>
> (Lees and Urwin 1991: 15)

What started out as a speech or language disorder in infancy and early childhood (see Case study 6.3) might well manifest later during the school years as a reading and writing problem, even after the original speech or language problem appears to have been successfully treated. This is because there is a close link between the processes involved in speech, language, spelling and reading (Stackhouse and Wells 1997), which all stem from the same underlying language system. When working with children who have problems with written language, it is advisable therefore to consider their understanding and use of spoken language, their speech and their phonological awareness skills (see page 146). Many childhood language disorders are life-long (Lees *et al*. 1991) and can affect the individual in different areas of life, such as making friends, completing school work and getting a job.

Disorders of language might be suspected in children who have delays in different aspects of their language system (for example, comprehension is good but expressive skills are poor) and whose language is developing in an unusual way (for example, more than usual difficulty retrieving words and using them appropriately, difficulty learning and using grammar including word endings, more than usual difficulty in learning how to use speech sounds to produce intelligible speech). There are many different ways that a language disorder may manifest, and one child's pattern of language impairment might be very different from another child's. It is very important to acknowledge that this type of disorder does not respond to 'generalized' language help, and therefore requires specialist support.

Neurological growth and development

Brain development is essential to the development of speech, language and communication skills, as to all areas of development. The brain sends messages to the articulators and the voice box and is where concept development, language processing and formulation and comprehension take place. Structural damage,

Case study 6.3 Tessa

Tessa is a 3-year-old girl who is receiving specialist support for her speech and language. As a baby she was often described as being in 'her own world' and would appear to 'switch off' now and again. She responded to her name much later than other children and did not start to babble until she was 11 months old. She attempted to point at interesting things when she was about 18 months using a splayed hand. She is interested in other people but does not usually initiate interactions with others, and needs a lot of support to keep interactions going.

Tessa's motor development is slightly slower than that of most other children the same age. She has and always has had normal hearing and her cognitive skills are considered to be within the range expected for her age. Her mother received some general advice about language stimulation, but found that this was not enough as Tessa was progressing very slowly with her language and speech. Tessa started making links between words and the things they represent towards the end of her second year. Her acquisition of language continues to be slow, and she finds some types of words extremely hard to learn. These include words like 'in' and 'under', which she learns more easily if there is visual information to support the spoken input.

dysfunction and slow maturation of the brain might all be implicated in difficulties with learning and developing communication skills (Kolb and Wishaw 1990). Genetic and environmental factors also contribute to how the brain develops (Mogford and Bishop 1993b). *Muscular dystrophy* (*Duchenne type*) and cerebral palsy carry a high risk of speech problems due to cerebral injury to speech mechanisms of the developing brain. This can affect the muscles necessary for respiration, voice and articulating speech. They can also impact on nonverbal communication expressed through facial expression, gesture and body language.

Although hard evidence of brain damage can be found in some children who have communication difficulties (for example, penetrating injury and cerebral bleeding), the majority of children with communication difficulties do not have these signs (Kolb and Wishaw 1990). Some have '*soft neurological signs*' such as attention disorders, motor clumsiness, hypoactivity or hyperactivity, poor body image, perceptual deficits, left–right problems and poor hand–eye coordination (Kolb and Wishaw 1990, Milloy and Morgan-Barry 1990) which are related to '*minimal brain dysfunction*'. This does not mean that there is any permanent damage to the brain, but that there is some problem in how it functions, and the way it functions can be inconsistent (Stock Kranowitz 1998).

It is necessary to consider whether children who have 'soft' neurological signs affecting motor skills or attention, for example, also have problems with their speech, language and communication. Many children who have significant

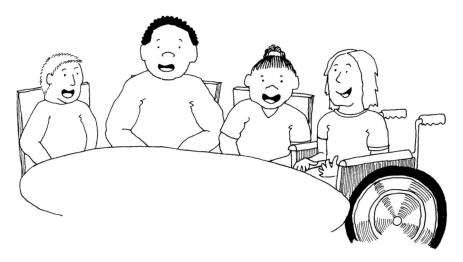

Figure 6.3 This physically disabled girl enjoys a conversation with her peers

difficulties with attention, for example, also have speech and language problems (Goldstein and Goldstein 1992) – some have additional difficulties 'reading' social situations and in responding to and using communication appropriately. Epilepsy is a marker of cerebral dysfunction and is present in many children with speech and language disorders (Robinson 1987), as is left-handedness or mixed-handedness, which indicates a difference in how the brain is developing relative to most other children. Such a difference does not necessarily imply there must be something wrong, however. There is increasing evidence of *cerebellar* involvement in specific language impairment and reading disorders (Tallal *et al.* 1993, Fawcett and Nicholson 1999).

Case study 6.4 Matthew

Matthew arrived for assessment of his communication skills with his mother just after his fourth birthday. It was hard for him to cross the room without tripping over. His speech was indistinct and it was hard to make sense of what he was saying some of the time. His attention kept drifting off. His mother was very worried because she had started noticing deterioration in Matthew's speech and language, in addition to other areas of his functioning (especially motor skills). She had expressed concerns to other professionals, but still did not know what was happening to her son. Matthew was eventually seen by a neurologist, who discovered that he had *hydrocephalus*, which required surgical intervention.

Structural growth and development

Children with physical difficulties affecting the structure or functioning of the lungs, voice box or articulators (see Figure I.2, page 7) might have problems developing speech, language and communication skills. *Cleft palate* and other structural anomalies affecting the face, articulators and vocal tract (see Figure I.3, page 7) usually impact directly on the development of speech, and are accompanied by a higher likelihood of hearing impairment.

When working with children who have speech difficulties related to an obvious physical cause, it is necessary to consider the child's overall speech, language and communication development, as less obvious language and communication difficulties can coexist with speech problems.

Sensory input: Hearing

Hearing impairment can have serious consequences on the development of speech, language and communication in children. Children might be born with a *sensorineural hearing loss* (resulting from damage to the hearing organ of the *inner ear* or damage along the sensory pathways that lead from the inner ear to the brain) or develop a hearing loss over the course of their development (usually affecting the middle part of the ear and frequently associated with a history of ear infections) (Northern and Downs 1984). Downs (1975) in Sancho *et al.* (1988) and Haggard (1992) estimate that 70 to 80 per cent of children between birth and 5 years have a hearing loss at any one time. For a proportion of children who suffer from *middle ear* difficulties affecting their hearing there can be long-term, damaging effects (Sancho *et al.* 1988, Hall 1989). There continues to be lack of appreciation among some professionals regarding the potential impact of mild but persistent hearing impairment on some children. This results in the children not receiving the right services at the right time to support their speech, language and communication skills. Hall (1989) suggests that screening for hearing impairment should take place for children who have:

- significantly impaired speech or language development
- chronic or repeated middle ear disease or upper airway obstruction
- developmental or behavioural problems.

Behavioural problems commonly arise in children who have *fluctuating hearing loss* resulting from *otitis media*, and who are often described as 'inattentive', 'distractible' and 'only responds to shouting'.

Hearing impairment arising from middle ear or inner ear problems results in difficulty perceiving the speech signal. The more severe impairments result in much slower acquisition of spoken language. Some compensation is afforded by visual cues but this is not usually adequate. Provided a visual communication system (for example sign language) is introduced early enough and occurs in a naturalistic context, children with severe hearing impairments will be able to communicate fluently, using that language.

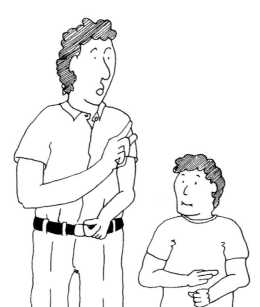

Figure 6.4 This hearing-impaired child and adult are using sign language to communicate

Case study 6.5 Patrick

Patrick was discovered to have profound hearing loss at the age of 4½. His family had outwardly resisted the possibility that there was anything amiss up until then, although his mother also had a profound hearing loss. There were concerns at school regarding his behaviour, as his main way of interacting with others was by pulling and tugging at people and grabbing things off them. His way of interacting with others improved markedly within six months after intensive help devoted to developing his verbal understanding and helping him to express himself, initially using signs.

Sensory input: Vision

Visual impairment may have some impact on the course of a child's language development, but usually has little impact on ultimate linguistic proficiency (Mogford and Bishop 1993b). There is typically some delay or difference relative to other children of the same age in speech and language development. This is thought to be related to differences in the establishment of joint attention (reduced or lack of eye gaze directing another person's attention towards something of interest, for example) and reduced learning of word meanings through seeing referents (the things the words refer to – toys, animals, people, actions, etc.) in context (Mogford and Bishop 1993b).

Case study 6.6 Sarah

Sarah, a 5-year-old with a severe visual impairment, had problems learning words denoting position, such as 'in front'. Sarah began to learn the meaning of these types of words by playing games with other children where they stood, jumped, and sat in front of (behind, next to, between) each other.

Risk factors associated with communication difficulties

Below is a list of risk factors associated with childhood communication difficulties (Paul 1995, Shipley and McAfee 1998):

- sensory impairments
- prematurity
- exposure to teratogens (foreign agents causing embryonic or fetal structural abnormalities) or infections in utero or during childhood
- maternal disease influencing normal growth of her unborn child
- birth trauma
- positive family history of communication difficulties
- medical and congenital conditions associated with communication impairments
- environmental deprivation and/or abnormal environmental input
- multiplicity of adverse factors.

Further reading

For further information on the range of childhood communication difficulties, readers are referred to the following texts:

Communication Difficulties in Childhood: A Practical Guide (1999) by James Law, Alison Parkinson and Rashmin Tamnhe (eds), Oxford: Radcliffe Medical Press.
Speech and Language Impairments in Children (2001) by Dorothy Bishop and L. Leonard (eds), New York: Psychology Press.
Diagnosis in Speech-language Pathology, 2nd edn (2000), by J. Tomblin, H. L. Morris and D.C. Spriestersbach (eds), San Diego, CA: Singular Publishing Group, Inc.
Time to Talk (2001) by M. Gloglowska, London: Whurr.
Children with Acquired Aphasias (1993) by J. Lees and B. Neville, London: Whurr.
Communication Disorders in Multicultural Populations (2001) by D. Battle, Burlington, MA: Butterworth-Heinemann.

Language Impairment and Psychopathology in Infants, Children and Adolescents (*Developmental Clinical Psychology and Psychiatry Paper 45*) (2001) by N. Cohen, London: Sage.

Developmental Speech and Language Disorders (1987) by D. Cantwell and L. Baker, New York, NY: Guilford Press.

Communication Disorders of Infants and Toddlers (1992) by F. Billeaud, Burlington, MA: Butterworth-Heinemann.

Paediatric Traumatic Brain Injury (1994) by R. DePompei and J. Blosser, San Diego, CA: Singular Publishing Group, Inc.

Communication Disorders and Children with Psychiatric and Behavioural Disorders (1998) by D. Rogers-Adkinson and P. Griffith (eds), San Diego, CA: Singular Publishing Group, Inc.

Craniofacial Anomalies (2000) by A. Kahn, San Diego, CA: Singular Publishing Group, Inc.

Acquired Neurological Speech and Language Disorders in Childhood (1990) by B. Murdoch (ed.), London: Taylor and Francis.

Communication Skills in Hearing-Impaired Children (1992) by J. Bench, London: Whurr.

Summary of Chapter 6

The nature of communication difficulties

1   Childhood communication difficulties are usually multi-factorial and are characterized by an interaction of environmental and internal factors.

2   Some childhood communication difficulties arise in association with other conditions affecting wider areas of a child's development, some occur in the absence of other developmental difficulties, and others are acquired over the course of childhood.

3   Communication difficulties might be due to development of communication skills that is delayed (i.e. following a normal pattern but at a slower pace) or disordered (i.e. following an unusual course).

Environmental and internal factors contributing to communication difficulties

4   Children usually develop normal communication skills in the context of reduced speech and language input, provided they experience 'normal human communication'.

5   Children of mothers who were depressed during the first few months of the baby's life are at risk of developmental difficulties, including delayed speech and language development.

6   Children's communication skills development is at risk if their experience of human communication is in the context of abusive or neglectful relationships with carers.

7   Children who have significantly reduced communication with others or lack of desire to communicate are at risk of developing communication disorders; some children use speech in some contexts but not in others, for example.

8   Children with abnormal social understanding and restricted knowledge of communication have difficulties relating to others and in using communication appropriately.

9   Children with impaired cognitive development, including those with general learning difficulties, usually have delayed (sometimes disordered) communication skills.

10 Many children have problems with speech and language processing in association with other developmental difficulties; some children have specific difficulty with their speech and language processing, however. This results in disordered speech and/or language development.

11 Structural damage, dysfunction and slow maturation of the brain, together with genetic and environmental influences on brain development, can impact on the development of communication skills.

12 Physical anomalies affecting verbal or nonverbal *output* can impact on the development of communication skills.

13 Hearing impairment can have a drastic effect on the development of communication skills, especially if children are not exposed to an appropriate communication system early enough.

14 Visual impairment usually entails development of communication skills along a different course, but this does not have a significant impact on communication skills in the long term.

15 All aspects of a child's developing communication system need to be carefully considered when any type of communication difficulty is suspected.

Working with parents of children with communication difficulties   **7**

- ○ Understanding parents of children with communication difficulties.
- ○ Models of parent–professional relationships; developing effective relationships.
- ○ Working with parents at different stages of their child's care.
- ○ Summary of key points.

Much of this chapter is relevant to professionals who work with parents of children with a wide range of developmental difficulties, including communication difficulties. However, since the focus of this book is on the development of communication in children, the focus of this chapter is on parents of children who have difficulties developing communication. This term is used to refer both to children whose communication difficulty is their main developmental problem (as in specific language impairment, described on pages 189–190), and to those whose communication difficulty is part of a wider developmental difficulty (as in a generalized learning difficulty, described on pages 188–189).

Which professionals?

Any professional who comes into contact with children during the course of their development is potentially in a position to identify a difficulty in the child's communication skills development. Some children's communication difficulties will be identified during infancy and the preschool years through health surveillance procedures and in preschool settings, and others will be identified during the school years. Some communication difficulties are not identified until adulthood, however.

Professionals who most commonly identify communication difficulties are health visitors and education staff such as early educators, educational psychologists and school teaching staff. Social workers, child-care providers, school nurses, general practitioners, paediatricians and audiological physicians are also well placed to observe children's communication skills, to talk with parents about any concerns they may have with regard to these and to make referrals for assessments by relevant agencies if indicated. In a parent survey conducted by AFASIC (Association for All Speech Impaired Children) (AFASIC 1993) looking at parents' experiences of services for their children with speech and language impairments, health visitors and general practitioners are the professionals to whom parents most commonly express initial concerns regarding their child's developing communication skills. Greater awareness of the development of communication skills in these two groups is essential.

Understanding parents of children with communication difficulties

Parents' feelings

Considering parents' feelings is central to working with them effectively in order to provide support for their child. It is the emotional bond between parents and children that is at the crux of parenting and which motivates parents to seek out explanations for differences in their child's development, and to help them.

Reactions to bad news

In suspecting and discovering that their child has a communication difficulty, many parents experience the full range of emotions associated with a grief response, in common with parents of children with other types of disabilities (Cunningham and Davis 1985, Lansdown 1980, Porter and McKenzie 2000). Characteristic stages of the grieving process have variously been recorded by writers over the years (Gross 1992). Perceptions that parents have of themselves and of their children might become invalidated through recognizing that their child has a disability (Cunningham and Davis 1985). In some cases, particularly those where children are identified as having life-long conditions such as learning difficulties and *autistic spectrum disorders*, parents may lose the image of the child they had envisaged having. They may need to reconstruct the image they have of themselves as parents, in addition to the one they have of their child. The extract 'Welcome to Holland' by Kingsley (undated) reproduced below from the Family Support Institute Newsletter goes some way towards illustrating this.

Welcome to Holland

When you're going to have a baby it's like you're planning a vacation to Italy. You're all excited. You get a whole bunch of guidebooks, you learn a few phrases in Italian so you can get around, and then it comes time to pack your bags and head for the airport – for Italy.

Only when you land, the flight attendant says 'Welcome to Holland.' You look at one another in disbelief and shock, saying 'Holland? What are you talking about? I signed up for Italy!'

But they explain there's been a change of plans, and you've landed in Holland, and there you must stay. 'But I don't know anything about Holland! I don't want to stay!' you say.

But you do stay. You go out and buy some new guidebooks, you learn some new phrases and you meet people you never knew existed. The important thing is that you are not in a filthy, plague-infested slum full of pestilence and famine. You are simply in a different place than you had planned. It's a slower place than Italy, less flashy than Italy, but after you've been there a little while and you have a chance to catch your breath you begin to discover that Holland has windmills. Holland has tulips. Holland has Rembrandts.

But everyone else you know is busy coming and going from Italy. They're all bragging about what a great time they had there and for the rest of your life you will say, 'Yes, that's what I had planned.'

The pain of that will never, ever go away. You have to accept that pain, because the loss of that dream, the loss of that plan, is a very, very significant loss. But if you spend your life mourning the fact that you didn't get to Italy, you will never be free to enjoy the very special, the very lovely things about Holland.

On receiving bad news from professionals with respect to their child's communication skills development, parents might experience shock, which can last for minutes or days. At such a time parents may be at their most vulnerable and in strong need of emotional support. They might go on to experience disbelief and deny the reality of what they have been told about their child. Disbelief might last several years, or just a few hours. Parents might experience a period of looking around for alternative explanations for their child's difficulty through seeking a second opinion, for example. They might find it very hard to acknowledge the bad news, as this would force an acknowledgement of the loss implicit in the bad news, which can be very hard. Anger may accompany or follow disbelief, and may be directed at professionals who have had some involvement in bringing the bad news. It is important to remember that, in most cases, anger is motivated by the diagnosis, not the individual professional. A period of despair might then follow, characterized by deep sorrow, uncontrollable weeping and morose thinking as anguish and pain become overwhelming. Reactions by parents to bad news in the form of disbelief, anger, denial, resentment and despair accompanied by feelings of sorrow, loss, anxiety, guilt and protectiveness are suggested by Cunningham and Davis (1985) and with other grief theorists to be evidence that they are exploring the situation, which is a necessary prerequisite to accepting it. Adaptation to and acceptance of the situation might be signalled by questions such as 'What can be done?' and 'What can we do to help?' Lansdown (1980) observes that at this, the final stage in the grief process, a sense of perspective returns with worry being under some control. This does not mean, however, that life is not problematic, nor that stages will not recur now and again in the future.

Professionals need to be aware of the possible emotional state of parents at various stages, as it is these feelings that help the process of adaptation to accept their situation (Cunningham and Davis 1985). Cunningham and Davis suggest that careful and well-organized counselling should be considered, to assist some parents through the process of adapting to their situation. They state that although parents' reactions may alter, their underlying emotions may last a long time and some may never be resolved. Of course, there is a wide variety of communication difficulties that different children have, and many can be overcome during childhood. Professionals need to recognize that parents are all different and will react to, and feel differently about, the news that their child has a communication difficulty, and that no assumptions can be made with regards to this.

Uncertainty about the future

In adapting to the situation, parents develop a greater understanding of their child's needs. This understanding helps to reduce anxiety and uncertainty about the child's current and future progress, although parents will almost always have questions about the future of their child, and there might always be an element of uncertainty, at least. Parents of children with communication difficulties ask many different types of questions. They ask about the likelihood of their child being able to talk at all, being able to hold a conversation, being able to meet their parent's eye gaze, being able to understand a simple joke, being able to understand their own and other people's emotions, being able to develop enough language to make and keep friends, being able to manage their anxiety, being able to control frustrated or aggressive behaviour, being able to learn the rules of conversation so other people do not get bored and give up, being able to say how they feel; they ask about the likelihood of their child going to a mainstream school, getting a job and establishing close emotional relationships later in life . . . The list is endless and as varied as the children, their parents and the types of communication difficulty facing them.

Guilt

Guilt is described by Lansdown (1980) as 'a slippery subject, hard to define exactly, difficult to discuss with parents until one knows them well, and even then not easy to pin down'. Cunningham and Davis (1985) define guilt as 'the awareness of a discrepancy between one's behaviour and one's own expectations of oneself'. Guilt is thought to exist when:

- parents consider their actions to have been in some way responsible for the child's developmental difficulty
- parents feel they have not done enough or sought help in good time for their child
- they lack knowledge about what to do
- they feel they are not doing enough for the rest of the family because of the particular needs of one child

- the child's condition is known to be inherited and the parents suspected a risk but did nothing to find out more.

Against these reasons, Cunningham and Davis and Lansdown warn against assuming parental guilt exists for the overly simplistic reason that they have produced a child who has a developmental difficulty or for 'allowing' a child to get ill. Parents of children with a communication skills difficulty frequently ask if their child's difficulty is due to something that they have done or not done. They need reassurance that it is not their behaviour that has brought about their child's difficulty, and to know that they are central to making a difference to their child's developing communication skills through supporting them.

Distress

Of course, children's communication difficulties are hugely varied – children who receive the same diagnosis often differ enormously in terms of how they are functionally and emotionally affected. It is also true that there is no one-to-one relationship between the severity of a child's developmental difficulty and the levels of distress experienced by their parents (Lansdown 1980). Professionals might be surprised at apparently low levels of distress expressed by parents of a child with severe language delay and high levels of distress expressed by parents of a child with mildly immature pronunciation.

Health and relationships

There is evidence that parents of children with developmental difficulties, especially those with learning difficulties, have higher rates of mental and physical ill health (Lansdown 1980). Lansdown also reports that while there is undoubtedly an added strain on the relationship between parents, 'the good marriages are made better and the bad ones worse'.

Positive feelings

There is little report in the literature of positive feelings expressed by parents of children with special needs, including communication difficulties. This is possibly because the relevant questions have not been asked, or if they have, have not been written up in the way that answers to questions about negative feelings have been. Of course, this should not lead to the assumption that these parents do not experience positive feelings just like any other parent, however, nor that they do not celebrate their child's successes and progress like other parents do.

The invisibility of many communication difficulties

Many parents of children with communication difficulties have to deal with the invisibility of their child's difficulty which can affect vast areas of their lives, including how they conduct their and their children's social lives, how they deal with being in public and how they and their children are perceived and understood by professionals. The National Autistic Society (UK) produces small cards which provide a brief description of autism for parents to give out as necessary to members of the public when out with their autistic child. This can help diffuse difficult situations that arise through the autistic child's behaviour and other people's reactions to it. As with many childhood communication difficulties, there are no outward physical signs of autism.

Invisibility of many communication difficulties can lead to misunderstandings among peers and adults regarding underlying reasons for a child's behaviour. Some children have subtle communication difficulties which impact on how they relate to other people and their ability to understand and use language and communication in the same ways other children of the same age do (see Chapter 6 for further details on childhood communication difficulties). Case study 7.1 illustrates how this type of communication difficulty may manifest.

Case study 7.1 Maria

Maria was a puzzle to many who knew her. At the age of 6 many of her sentences were very well formed and 'adult-like'. She knew many stories off by heart, and recited extracts of these on occasion. Maria preferred adult company, and she impressed many adults with her apparently 'good' language skills. However, her teachers reported that something was 'not quite right' about Maria. She used to ask many questions, but did not really show interest in the answers given, she would 'take over' conversations, showed little idea about turn-taking, and favoured particular topics. She would get distressed quickly when given directions at school, and had difficulty understanding abstract words, in particular those relating to time, such as 'yesterday', 'soon', 'before' and so on. She sometimes made up words without being aware she had done so, and frequently used words incorrectly. Maria found it hard to form close friendships and she tended to dominate play with peers. Her parents were very reluctant to agree to Maria's teacher referring her for assessment of her communication skills. It was only after two years at school, when her academic progress was slower than expected, that this referral took place. Assessment of Maria's language revealed a very uneven profile of abilities. Her verbal comprehension was much lower than her parents had thought, she had great difficulty selecting correct words to name pictures and had problems explaining things. Her ability to recite long extracts from stories was due to Maria's good memory for things she had heard and seen, but her understanding of much spoken language was, however, very poor.

Daniel's mother describes an event that occurred when Daniel, who had a subtle communication disorder, was 7:

> It was sports day and all the children were in a race together. The race involved a number of items such as coloured hoops and skittles and string baskets. The object of the exercise was to pick up a hoop and run to the nearest basket and drop it in, run back and pick up another then run to the next basket (further down the course) and drop it in. This process was carried out until the last item was dropped into the basket at the terminal end of the course. From there the children ran all the way back to the starting point. Daniel did not seem to have grasped the fact that it was a competition, and was being very tidy in putting all the items in the baskets (his and those of his competitors) that had missed. His pace lacked any urgency, contrasting quite starkly with all the other children in the race. It provoked laughter from all the parents watching, but Daniel did not know that he was doing anything wrong.

This is a poignant example of how misunderstood some communication disorders are. There was no outward sign that Daniel had a communication disorder and other people, including his teachers, repeatedly misunderstood his behaviour as they did not realize the extent to which he was unable to follow verbal instructions, missed the point of many events and activities and had limited understanding of communication generally. He was regularly described as 'awkward' and 'difficult', especially by staff at his secondary school who did not understand his problems and by whom Daniel now feels let down. Daniel's mother had to fight a 'long hard battle' to get his difficulties and needs recognized by school staff. It was due to her commitment to her son and sense of knowing that something was wrong that he was finally seen at the age of 7 by an educational psychologist who recommended specialist help, which he eventually got. There are countless examples of parents with concerns about their children's communication difficulties not being taken seriously by professionals (AFASIC 1993), resulting in their children's developmental needs not being met, often with long-term consequences for their chances in life, and in parents experiencing high levels of stress and anxiety.

Daniel's brother, James, was born with a moderate sensori-neural hearing loss. Although this was not identified until he was 3 (and through a friend, initially), professionals then put his mother in touch with relevant support organizations and gave her appropriate information with which to help her son. Against significant limitations, James has subsequently progressed very well, a fact which his mother attributes to the levels and appropriateness of the support which he has received. James and Daniel's mother suggests that it is due to the more 'concrete' nature of hearing impairment that James' needs were identified and subsequently met in a way which Daniel's were not.

Reactions by others

Other people's attitudes towards disability, particularly in children, can contribute to making parents of children with developmental difficulties, including communication difficulties, feel different from other families (Lansdown 1980). This can lead to social isolation, which might be reduced by placing such families in touch with other families who have similar problems. A list of useful contacts is included at the back of this book (page 222), which may be of use to parents of children who have communication difficulties. Many people who are unfamiliar with differences in how people look, behave and communicate might be fearful of these differences, and a barrier can be created by their fear. An increase in knowledge about a particular disability is usually accompanied by a reduction in fear and an increase in sensitivity.

Other problems

Financial

As with any parent of a child with a developmental difficulty, parents of children with communication difficulties may find themselves financially worse off due to various factors, such as one parent stopping work in order to look after their child and coordinate their care from the different services and professionals. They might have to meet transport costs of travelling to and from hospital or clinic appointments, and in some cases to and from specialist resource centres and schools. Private health care might be chosen by some families due to limited resources in their area, particularly for therapy services.

Social life and support system

Parents might not be able to find babysitters who can manage the particular needs of some children with communication difficulties, thus affecting their social lives. They might be reluctant to leave their child in the care of another person, for fear of what might happen. Family members, friends and associates of parents are reported in some cases to avoid the parents around the time of their child's diagnosis, resulting in fragmentation of their support system.

Siblings

By the time they are 11, five out of six children have a sibling (Lansdown 1980). About two-thirds of the brothers and sisters of children with developmental difficulties who have been studied were shown to cope without showing undue strain. Lansdown summarizes what is known about the problems of the other third of siblings:

- Children who are younger than the child with developmental difficulties are more vulnerable, especially to anxiety (Coleby 1995); near-age siblings had less contact with peers.
- Girls are more vulnerable than boys; older male siblings had greater appreciation for the child with disabilities, while older female siblings showed more behavioural problems – possibly related to being over-burdened with child-care responsibilities (Coleby 1995).
- Most disturbances are found in siblings of children with life-threatening, inherited conditions; all too frequently they have not received adequate information and fear that they or their children might get the condition.
- Jealousy, attention-seeking behaviour and regression might all be evident in siblings.
- Although siblings might be loving, tender and protective towards the child at home, they might be acutely embarrassed in public, get teased at school and not bring friends home.

The implications of these findings are that many parents of children with developmental difficulties, including communication difficulties, have even more to cope with in their families than might be expected. They need to balance parenting to ensure that the sibling of a child with special needs does not permanently feel they are 'second place' (Trachtenberg and Batshaw 1997). Siblings are reported as often showing increased maturity, sense of responsibility and tolerance of 'being different'; many ultimately enter helping professions (Trachtenberg and Batshaw 1997). For further reading on young carers, including those caring for a disabled sibling, see Chace (2000).

Vulnerability to maltreatment

Research has shown that premature infants and low birthweight babies and children with some developmental difficulties (learning difficulties and physical disabilities) are more vulnerable than other children to parental maltreatment (Hetherington and Parke 1986). Many of these children are very fussy, difficult to soothe, cry excessively with a particularly irritating cry and may have physical needs and differences which contribute to the parents feeling antagonistic towards the child. Culp *et al.* (1991) cite Martin (1976) who notes that these are characteristics that make caring for a child difficult or unrewarding. Martin also proposed that children with milder disabilities might be most vulnerable to parental maltreatment as their problems might be more difficult to detect and associated assistance from professionals might not be forthcoming. Culp *et al.* (1991) also cite other writers who speculate that children with language difficulties might fall into this bracket of most vulnerable, in that their limited language skills could make caring for the child difficult, and could result in unrewarding conversations and interactions. Further research is needed to investigate any relationship that might exist between subtle disabilities such as language disability and increased likelihood of parental maltreatment, as there is very little covering this area.

Parent–professional relationships

The key point underpinning this section is the fact that outcomes for children are significantly improved when parents are supported effectively and sensitively and involved in their children's management and their programmes (Lansdown 1980, Porter and McKenzie 2000). Porter and McKenzie cite research stating that parental involvement, whether in early intervention or later transition from schooling to adult life, is the main determinant of success. These facts (which are hopefully obvious to most professionals at the current time) have been learned as a result of several changes over the years in the parent–professional relationship.

There has been increasing contact between parents and professionals over the years, due partly to an increase in understanding about special needs, with a consequent improvement in services (Cunningham and Davis 1985). Before exploring this area further, it is necessary to think about what parents and professionals respectively bring to the care of a child with a developmental difficulty.

What is a parent, and what is a professional?

These questions are answered below with respect to the care of a child with a developmental difficulty. The answers draw on the work of Porter and McKenzie (2000), Cunningham and Davis (1985) and Lansdown (1980).

A parent is:

- the child's legal guardian
- the child's main advocate
- the person who has the right to make reasonable and unreasonable demands on behalf of their child
- the person who makes decisions in the child's interests
- the person who provides professionals with information on the child's needs, wishes and preferences
- the person who must balance the child's needs with those of the other members of the family
- the person who involves professionals when their help is required and from whom they expect honesty and accuracy
- the person who has expert knowledge of the child and their home environment
- the person who is thoroughly committed to the child
- the person who has a high emotional involvement with the child
- the person who has direct experience of having a child with special needs.

A professional is:

- the person with specialist knowledge on child development and disability
- the person with knowledge of relevant services and of how to gain access to these
- the person who has a short-term commitment to the child and the family

- the person who must listen to what the parents say about their child and recognize limitations in their professional knowledge and competence
- the person who must make onward referrals when needed to other services when they recognize that a child's or family's needs extend beyond their own role
- the person who must offer a service that promotes the interests of the child and family, balanced with their responsibilities to their employer and the wider community.

Evolving models of the parent–professional relationship

In order that everybody is able to work towards promoting the child's development and thus securing better outcomes for them in all aspects of life, it is necessary that a trusting, honest and cooperative relationship exists between professionals and parents (Cunningham and Davis 1985). Taking account of the information about their children that most parents are able to provide and their high levels of motivation to care for their child, and taking account of the skills and knowledge that professionals have at their disposal, anybody would have to conclude that the best outcomes for children are achieved through partnership between parents and professionals between whom there exists a two-way need. How that partnership is realized has been the subject of change and development over the years, the course of which is briefly outlined below.

Professionals as experts

In the past, lay people viewed professionals as having high status by virtue of their specialist knowledge, and deferred to their opinions (Porter and McKenzie 2000). Parents of children with developmental difficulties were regarded by professionals as being peripheral to those children's needs, resulting in residential institutionalization of many such children. Despite advances in how disability is viewed and the relative roles of parents and professionals, there remain proponents of the 'professional as expert' model, perhaps unwittingly in some cases. Parents are only given as much information as the professional deems relevant. Daniel's mother (see page 204) never received a diagnosis for her son until a chance encounter in a supermarket with a professional who had previously worked with him (by this time Daniel was 20, had dropped out of college and was unable to get a job, largely due to factors which his mother and others who know him well link to his communication disorder). During the course of the conversation, the professional 'let slip' Daniel's diagnosis, thus opening the flood-gates of information for his mother to which she had never previously been privy. In recounting her experiences, Daniel's mother recalls that the professionals involved with her son had 'not liked labels'. (The issue of diagnosis is discussed in more detail on pages 215–218.) Daniel's mother commented,

I felt devastated. How could they sit on that diagnosis and not fill me in and help me with things at home. Just because they didn't like to use labels. I got my education, but a bit late.

Her chance encounter with the professional in question occurred in 2001.

Lack of parental involvement by professionals is linked to high levels of dissatisfaction, incomplete or inaccurate understanding, reluctance to question the professional and low levels of cooperation on the part of parents (Cunningham and Davis 1985). Parents might become overly dependent on the professionals, giving rise to an increasing sense of inadequacy and incompetence. Cunningham and Davis point out that professionals who do not seek out parental views on children they work with run the risk of limiting their understanding of those children to one determined solely by their own professional framework. This can lead to missing important problems the child has and ignoring additional elements in the child's physical and social environment that could otherwise be used as resources in the child's support programme.

Transferral of knowledge and skills

All professions have developed towards this model (Cunningham and Davis 1985), which views parents as relevant to children's intervention while the professional maintains control over making decisions about long- and short-term aims of intervention and methods used. Professionals continue to view themselves as having expertise but also view parents as a resource. Knowledge and skills possessed by professionals are channelled over to parents to use with their children. Wider aspects of the child's life and therefore other problems encountered are less likely to be missed by professionals, and parents are less likely to suffer from low self-confidence and are better able to make necessary adjustments.

Inherent in this model of the parent–professional relationship is the risk of viewing parents as a homogenous group (Cunningham and Davis 1985) with equal amounts of energy, resources, motivation, time and understanding of what is expected of them. Parents may not share the same views as the professional regarding intervention aims and may disagree with methods used. Increasing numbers of speech and language therapists treat preschool children who have delayed communication skills by supporting their parents' interaction skills and raising parents' awareness of how their interaction with their child impacts on the child's speech and language development. Programmes are planned for individuals and groups of parents with many reports of positive outcomes for both children and parents (Girolametto *et al.* 1996a, Girolametto *et al.* 1996b, Weitzman 1996, Watson 1998). However, this type of intervention is not appropriate for all children, nor indeed for all parents who may not welcome or find value in such methods.

Collaboration

A collaborative model of working recognizes an equivalent balance of power between parents and professionals, acknowledges parents' areas of expertise and reinforces their rights. Collaboration occurs when parents and professionals share responsibility for gathering relevant information and jointly plan and evaluate intervention targets (Friend and Cook 1996, cited by Porter and McKenzie 2000). In addition to providing professional knowledge and skills, the professional provides parents with relevant information regarding available resources, services and intervention methods to help them decide how best to make use of these in order to help their child. Professionals and parents engage in a process of negotiation during which the professional's role is to 'listen and understand the parent's views, aims, expectations, current situation and resources . . . to help the parents to reach realistic and effective decisions' (Cunningham and Davis 1985). The professional's role is to support parents in their chosen role (Porter and McKenzie 2000), which may involve a greater or lesser amount of active involvement by them.

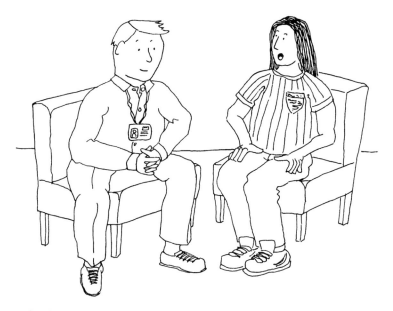

Figure 7.1 Discussion between a professional and a parent

Implications for effective working

The fact that professionals are being consulted by parents at all usually indicates a desire for some change for the child and family – professionals must respond by listening and with the intention of helping. Complaints that parents have made about services from professionals have focused on the following areas: poor communication, perceived lack of warmth and compassion, competence, availability of resources, accessibility of services, poor organization of services, inefficient liaison between professionals, lack of continuity in a child's care and ineffectiveness (Cunningham and Davis 1985). Some of these points will be considered here. There needs to be effective communication between parents and professionals, including clarity regarding their expectations of each other, and therefore of the parent–professional relationship. This is necessary in order to avoid misconceptions and uncertainty, build confidence and trust and enable the sharing of expertise. There needs to be a recognition of the complementary nature of parent and professional roles and a pooling of each other's knowledge, experience and skills. Cunningham and Davis additionally call for professionals to have specific training in how to establish effective relationships with parents in order that their specialist skills can be implemented fully. Porter and McKenzie (2000) observe that many parents of children with special needs encounter several professionals over the child's lifetime and therefore have varied experiences of the parent–professional relationship. Some might have felt let down by 'the system' and by services and lose trust in professionals' competence and skills. The need for professionals to be aware of the limitations and boundaries of their knowledge and expertise is underscored with regard to these issues.

Considerations for working with parents at different stages of their child's care

Considering the following questions should help professionals to develop effective relationships with parents of children with communication difficulties at each stage of a child's care, and thus increase the likelihood of improving the child's outcomes:

- What do her parents need?
- What is the purpose of my involvement currently with regards to meeting her parents' needs?
- What can I do to help her parents support their child's communication skills?

Summers *et al.* (1990), in Porter and McKenzie (2000), Bibbings (1994) and Cunningham and Davis (1985) state between them that what parents of children with developmental difficulties need at each stage in their child's care is:

- information to enable them to help their child effectively
- for them and their child to be dealt with competently
- practical support wherever possible
- emotional and psychological support.

With regards to providing emotional support, Porter and McKenzie (2000) recommend that professionals relate to parents in a natural way rather than adopting a formal 'professional' role.

Identifying communication difficulties

In 1986, Enderby and Phillip stated that up to half a million children in the UK of preschool or school age were expected to have a communication difficulty at some point. In 1998 the NHS Centre for Reviews and Dissemination claimed that 6 in 100 children will have a speech, language or communication difficulty at some point in their lives; Hall (1996) identified that at least 1 in 500 children experiences severe, long-term communication difficulties.

Parents are experts on their children and as such are best placed to provide information which will help in the identification of any difficulty in their child's communication skills development. Several different circumstances may lead to a meeting between parents and professionals during which one or the other expresses concern about a child's communication skills. Many parents of children with communication difficulties will know from the birth of their child that there is a problem, as in the case of congenitally deaf babies whose hearing impairment has been identified due to appropriate use of screening procedures. Some parents identify communication difficulties in their children and seek out an explanation from professionals and are successful in obtaining an onward referral for assessment of the child's communication skills.

However, many parents may not know for sure for many months or even years that there is a problem. By the time they take their child for an assessment of their communication skills, some parents may have suspected for a long time that something was wrong but have not been taken seriously by those to whom they previously voiced concerns. A parent survey looking at parents' experience of services offered to children with speech and language impairments found that although parents are the ones to recognize their child's difficulty in the majority of cases, 'the experience of many parents is that they find it difficult to persuade professionals to take their concerns seriously' (AFASIC 1993). Among the major issues raised and outlined in this report is the need for earlier diagnosis and help for speech and language impairment, especially in the preschool years.

Some parents, however, may not agree that their child has difficulty developing their communication skills, for a variety of reasons notably including lack of knowledge regarding normal language development (Hall 1996). Hall suggests that many parents, including highly educated ones, may benefit from guidance and information on language development in an accessible form. Health visitors are well placed to provide information on language development in health education sessions to parenting groups, mother and baby groups and postnatal groups.

Inadequate knowledge about the development of communication skills, and the nature of communication itself are two factors that contribute to the variation in when and how children's communication skills are eventually identified.

Inadequate knowledge

There is inadequate knowledge amongst parents and professionals about the development of communication skills, especially during infancy. In AFASIC's parent survey (AFASIC 1993), the first sign of communication difficulty was noticed (by parents, in 83 per cent of cases) before intelligible speech is expected – that is to say from birth to approximately 18 months. The signs noticed included:

- no infant babbling
- no early speech sounds
- baby did not cry
- constant crying
- unusual eye contact
- child withdrawn and silent
- feeding difficulties.

On early signs of a difficulty in Daniel's development, his mother comments,

> It was certainly my experience that Daniel had problems with feeding as an infant. The distress, rejection and frustration I felt at Daniel's inability to breast feed have remained with me ever since. He was an uncooperative, unresponsive, miserable baby who contrasted dramatically with babies of friends. Even if he wasn't intentionally neglected or mistreated, I do think he missed some love along the way as a result of his communication difficulties.

However, despite early recognition by parents in the AFASIC survey, fewer than 2 out of 3 children had received help by the age of 4 years, and only 2 out of 3 had received a diagnosis by the age of 5 years. What is not clear is (1) the extent to which parents who recognize early signs of a communication difficulty wait (in some cases several months, or years) before expressing concerns to a professional, compared against (2) the extent to which parents who recognize early signs of a difficulty are not taken seriously by professionals they express concerns to. Either way, the result is that many children with developmental communication difficulties are not referred early enough to a suitably qualified professional who is able to give an appropriate diagnosis. It remains within the remit of professionals to look out for difficulties in all areas of a child's development, and respond to parents' concerns appropriately. The principles of inter-professional and inter-agency working in the best interests of the child are enshrined in legislation in the UK (The Children Act 1989) and in guidelines for assessment of children and families (for example The Assessment Framework, Department of Health 1999). They are at the heart of community-based initiatives in the UK that support vulnerable families with young children in order to give the children a better chance in life (Sure Start Unit 2002).

The nature of communication and development of these skills

Communication and the development of communication skills is generally taken for granted and it is not until there is evidence of a difference or a breakdown in communication that we are forced to analyse it. Even then, differences in communication are subject to individual parents' and, in many cases, professionals' perceptions of what is normal and abnormal communication. Unlike tangible differences such as the absence of a limb, blindness or paralysis, most childhood communication difficulties are invisible, as discussed earlier. (See Chapter 6 for information on the range of childhood communication difficulties.) Also, many communication difficulties are multi-factorial in nature and might involve difficulties in understanding or using language, in articulating speech due to physical limitations or in hearing auditory input adequately as in hearing impairment.

Although there may be an outward sign in some children of a communication difficulty, such as a hearing aid or a surgically repaired cleft lip and palate, it can be hard for the untrained observer to detect the true range and level of communication impairment as many 'obvious' difficulties will be accompanied by invisible ones. For example, children with clefts might also have slower language development and are more susceptible to fluctuating hearing loss than other children of the same age. These factors have contributed to many children's speech, language and communication needs not being identified by professionals until school age (AFASIC 1993), sometimes not until early adulthood, and in some cases not at all.

How can professionals try to ensure that children with communication difficulties are appropriately identified?

Many points are raised below in answer to this question. Although it is not always possible for all professionals to do everything highlighted below, an awareness of these factors, at least, is fundamental to the establishment of an effective parent–professional relationship.

- Listen to parents and take their concerns about their children's development, including their communication skills, seriously. This might include taking appropriate action to refer to relevant services for an assessment of a child's communication skills and/or other areas of development. If there is a parental or professional concern regarding a child's communication skills development, an assessment by a suitably qualified speech and language therapist is indicated.
- Update your knowledge and/or gain access to reliable sources of information regarding what communication skills to expect in children at different ages.
- Be honest with parents and talk through any concerns in a sensitive and open way. Professionals need to use their knowledge of the child and their knowledge of child development, in particular of communication skills development when substantiating their reasons for raising concerns. Striking a balance between not bombarding parents with information yet not omitting necessary information is important in order to communicate a clear picture of professional concern to parents.
- Obtain relevant information on the child's abilities and performance in different contexts, including at home (Porter and McKenzie 2000).
- Don't pre-empt a diagnosis if not suitably qualified (Porter and McKenzie 2000).

- Know what relevant services are available locally, their referral procedures and criteria, waiting times, and what type of service a family might expect to receive.
- Communicate this information to parents, so they have realistic expectations of local services and are less likely to feel let down before they have started seeking help.
- Provide additional relevant information to parents, such as details of local or national support groups, charities and other organizations which can help and inform parents of children who might have a developmental difficulty (see 'Useful Addresses', page 222). However, it is important to judge timing of providing this type of information carefully. For some parents it might be better to wait until a later stage in the child's care.
- Be sensitive to a parent's emotional state when discussing their child's development and needs, and be prepared for a variety of reactions, including resistance, shock, relief and gratefulness.
- Maintain effective liaison with relevant professionals from local services and understand each other's roles.
- Provide adequate information to relevant services when making referrals for children suspected of having communication difficulties, in order to help with prioritization. The type of information and level of detail required can be obtained through a process of liaison with those services.
- Provide parents with practical assistance where appropriate and possible. This might include helping with filling out forms, working out how to get to the appointment, accompanying parents to the appointment and providing information on obtaining interpreting services if relevant.
- Remember that it really is better to be safe than sorry when there is a concern expressed regarding a child's development, including their communication skills. Professionals would prefer to see a child and discharge them rather than risk missing a difficulty of some kind.
- Plan the meeting very carefully, and respond very carefully to parents' expressions of concerns. This can be achieved by leaving enough time for discussion and for listening to parents' perceptions and reactions.
- Avoid 'casually killing dreams' (Porter and McKenzie 2000) parents might have developed about their children, themselves as parents and the family in general.

Diagnosis of a communication difficulty

Why diagnose?

There are negative and positive aspects to giving children diagnoses, and there exist differences within groups of professionals and parents on the relative merits of diagnosing and not diagnosing.

Professionals cannot always be certain of diagnoses when formulating opinions about children. Some diagnoses are made on the basis of a child's behaviour at one point in their lives, and a history of their behaviour. Some of these children might receive a different diagnosis at a later stage in their development. Negative connotations of a diagnosis may impact on parents' perceptions of their child's current skills and likely ability to progress.

Deferred diagnoses, for children with severe and complex communication disorders, that can occur when professionals are not certain, have been found to result in far greater parental stress than providing a 'working', or 'provisional' diagnosis (appropriate for when professionals are mostly, but not completely, certain) (Filipek and Prizant 1999, Filipek and Prizant 2000). Some parents of children who eventually received a diagnosis of autistic spectrum disorder were found to have waited between six months and two years (Prizant 2001). Prizant (2001) reports that the combination of an 'invisible' disability and uncertainty about diagnosis leads to greater stress levels in parents. The parent survey undertaken by AFASIC (1993) reported that two-thirds of children with speech and language impairment were not given a diagnosis by the first professional they saw, but had received one by the time they were 5. Nearly all the remaining one-third received a diagnosis during their infant or junior school years; only 1 in 200 children reached the age of 12 without a diagnosis. Reasons given in the report for certain diagnoses being made later than others include the possibility that such diagnoses can be made with greater confidence at a later stage in the child's development. However, it is worth noting that these are usually in cases of more complex and lower incidence communication disorders requiring the expertise of speech and language therapists and paediatricians. Some comments on the subject of obtaining a diagnosis from parents included in that report follow:

> It has taken over three years to get a diagnosis, and this has only come about by myself being determined to find out more. Paediatricians should refer problem children on, surely, not just say they are clueless?
>
> We felt that we were floundering around for over a year, waiting to see someone, not sure we were seeing the right person and being told to wait until he was older to see if there was a problem.
>
> Things should move more quickly – it takes so much badgering and bullying to get things moving, and your child is getting older and older.

In spite of the potentially negative effects of labels on the individuals who receive them (to do with professional uncertainty regarding diagnosis and potential negative impact on parental perceptions of the child), many parents find diagnostic labels helpful in understanding their children's needs, difficulties and behaviour. Labels can be useful in describing, explaining and predicting (in some cases) children's developmental progress (Porter and McKenzie 2000). Early diagnosis is associated with motivating families to seek support and is the first step in early intervention, which is related to better outcomes for children (Prizant 2001).

How can professionals help parents at the time of diagnosis?

Once again, there are practical limitations regarding what professionals can be realistically expected to do with regards to helping parents, but awareness of the following points is important.

- Provide information on the child's condition, possible causes, treatments available and prognosis, wherever possible. Encourage questions, answer them and guide parents to reliable sources of information for answers to questions that they cannot answer. Be honest about the current state of professional knowledge regarding a child's difficulty at the present time and their likely future development.
- Provide the information in different ways and at different times during the meeting, and avoid the use of technical terms and confusing language.
- Ensure adequate time is given to parents when giving a diagnosis, in order that they may ask questions. Some professionals may wish to tape record the meeting and give parents the tape to take home, as it can be difficult for parents to retain all the information discussed in such a meeting and to recount it to a partner afterwards. Offer a second meeting, to take place soon after the first, to allow for further discussion and questions once the initial news has sunk in.
- Provide practical assistance and jointly devise strategies to help parents help their children at the present time wherever possible. Many parents of language delayed children welcome advice on stimulating language development, for example.
- Provide information on any benefits the family might be eligible for, and on relevant services in the area and how to access these.
- Provide emotional and psychological support, and be prepared for a range of reactions from parents to the diagnosis. Guide parents towards appropriate sources of support and avoid making assumptions about their emotional state and reactions to the situation on a short- or a long-term basis.
- Remember that parents might be at their most vulnerable around the time their child's difficulty is identified, and consider carefully how parents may wish to be related to at this time.
- Respond to all parents as individuals, regardless of their cultural backgrounds.
- Acquaint yourself with cultural values of families from other cultures, in particular regarding social cooperation, competition, academic success, disability and social-emotional development (Porter and McKenzie 2000). Use this knowledge to consider what expectations families from other cultures might have of services, and thus how effectively these will be used to support their child's developmental difficulty.
- Provide parents with information on local and national organizations, charities and parent support groups as appropriate to their and their child's needs, when parents express an interest in taking up such contacts.
- Avoid overwhelming parents with information and potentially helpful contacts; be guided by them regarding how much information to provide, and when.

- Don't omit negative information out of the desire to protect parents (Porter and McKenzie 2000). Maintain sensitivity and tact.
- Be aware of your own attitudes towards disability and how these might impinge on the relationship you have with parents, and the impression parents might receive regarding their child's disability.
- Understand parents' perceptions of relevant services and encourage use of services as appropriate.

After the diagnosis

Once a child's communication difficulty has been diagnosed, parents continue to need psychological and emotional support, information on how to help their child and practical assistance wherever possible. Suggestions for how professionals can support parents at this stage in their child's care can be found below.

A key issue that arises after parents become aware of their child's difficulty is education. Many children in the UK do not receive the level or type of educational support necessary to adequately support their communication needs (AFASIC 1993). One of the reasons underlying this relates to inconsistency within and among education authorities concerning how communication needs are viewed and thus how they are supported. Another reason is the dire shortage of qualified speech and language therapists in the UK. Parents frequently use words such as 'battle' and 'fight' when talking about the struggle they have had when endeavouring to get appropriate support for their child's communication needs (AFASIC 1993, Lorenz 1998, author's personal communication with parents).

How can professionals help parents after a diagnosis?

- Provide information on educational resources and how to access these.
- Support parents in their quest to obtain appropriate educational support for their child.
- Maintain effective liaison with all professionals involved in a child's care, seek to understand and explain to relevant others the educational implications of the child's communication difficulty and provide support in the educational setting as appropriate.
- Be aware of relevant legislation that might impact on securing a child appropriate educational support.
- Lorenz (1998) recommends that nurseries and schools work in partnership with parents of children with developmental difficulties through encouraging them to become active in the life of the school, meeting regularly, listening to their concerns and needs, involving them in their child's programme, keeping them informed of the professionals involved in their child and when visits take place, obtaining their views before changing provision, celebrating with them when progress is made, trusting them to cooperate if there are problems and valuing them as partners in the education of their child. She reminds professionals that

many parents will have more up-to-date information on their child's condition than some professionals, and strongly supports sharing teaching strategies and information with them.

- Encourage parents to maintain a sense of normality through contact with the outside world and provide practical information and advice to help them do so, particularly regarding child care, if parents want it.
- Help family members remain aware of each other's needs. Contact with other families in similar positions and relevant support organizations can be helpful in this respect (Lansdown 1980).
- Provide encouragement and support to parents to go to the proper sources for help, including respite help if needed.
- Help parents to decide what to tell their child about their difficulty, and what to tell other members of the family, if they want this type of help.
- Help parents think about how to manage difficult situations that might arise in public, if relevant, and if parents want this type of help.
- Try to understand parents' emotional reactions. Provide emotional and psychological support or information on where parents can get this type of support, if they want it. Recognize that some parents may experience recurring and even life-long feelings of grief and loss triggered by different events and stages in their child's life, and respond sensitively to these.
- Use professional knowledge, knowledge about services and one's understanding of the child and family to help parents plan realistically for the future.
- Look beyond the diagnosis in order to focus on the whole child and help parents do the same, if indicated. Share professional knowledge with parents to help them make sense of their child's behaviour, progress and abilities and help parents to continue to build their knowledge as their child develops and progresses.
- Help parents to focus on their child's current needs in order jointly to plan and deliver therapy or educational programmes effectively and reduce the risk of parents getting 'burned out'.
- Remember that the way a child's parents behave is 'crucial to the way the child copes with his condition' (Lansdown 1980).

Concluding remarks

Inspired by Lansdown (1980), this chapter concludes with a few thoughts relevant to professionals who work with parents of children with communication difficulties:

- Never say, 'Don't worry', as parents will and should worry at times.
- Never say 'I understand how you feel', unless you do.
- Do not assume parents will trust and respect you just because you are a professional. Dealing with parents and their children with honesty, sensitivity and competence will, however, help develop trusting, effective relationships between parents and professionals.

The combined efforts, knowledge, experiences and motivations of parents and professionals help children develop to their fullest potential. Promoting children's communication skills is most successful when undertaken as a joint responsibility by all those involved in a child's communication development. It is only by working through parents and other key adults in a child's life such as teachers that a functional approach to intervention is achieved, ensuring that the communication skills being taught are those that children need to know.

Professionals and parents alike know that the development of communication skills is fundamental to any child's development. A greater understanding of what these skills are, and of how and when they develop will lead to greater confidence in all parties regarding what to expect at different ages. This can only result in earlier identification of communication difficulties and thus earlier intervention, which is now widely acknowledged to be highly beneficial to children.

Summary of Chapter 7

Which professionals?

1   Any professional who works with young children is potentially in a position to identify difficulties in any aspect of their development, including their communication skills.
2   Greater knowledge and awareness of the development of communication skills in young children, especially in infancy, is needed in professionals who work with young children, particularly among health visitors and general practitioners.

Understanding parents of children with communication difficulties

3   Professionals need to be aware of, and therefore be prepared to respond sensitively to, the range of feelings and reactions that parents might experience at different stages of their child's care, and to recognize that parents' varying feelings help them to adapt to their situation.
4   Professionals should not make assumptions regarding how parents might feel at different stages of their child's care.
5   Professionals need to know that many childhood communication difficulties have no outward physical sign; some may be masked by apparently 'good' language skills or be accompanied by unusual behaviour, or behaviour that is beyond the realms of what would otherwise be expected in other children at the same stage of development.

Parent–professional relationships

6 Professionals need to listen to and take seriously any concerns that parents express regarding their child's developing communication skills.
7 Professionals need to know the limits of their own knowledge and experience with regards to the development of communication skills in children and seek the opinion, when indicated, of a speech and language therapist. Speech and language therapists are the only professionals who receive specific training in the assessment of children's communication skills.
8 Professionals need to be aware of the range of difficulties that might be faced by parents caring for a child with a communication difficulty, and take these into account in their work.
9 Outcomes for children are improved when parents are effectively and sensitively involved in their child's management and programmes.
10 Professionals need to be aware of the complementary nature of their and parents' relative areas of skill, knowledge and expertise.
11 Professionals need to know what their model of working is with parents, and to know how to develop effective communication with parents.

Considerations for working with parents at different stages of their child's care

12 Professionals need to remember that parents need information, practical assistance and emotional support at each stage of their child's care, to help them help their child.
13 There is a strong need for earlier identification of communication difficulties in infancy and the preschool years.
14 Professionals need to consider their views towards diagnosis of a child's developmental difficulties and how these might impact on a parent's understanding of their child's difficulties, on their motivation to seek appropriate help, on their need for information, practical assistance and psychological support.
15 Professionals need to consider how to deliver sensitively information to parents of children with communication difficulties at each stage of their child's care.
16 Where relevant, professionals need to consider how they can help parents obtain appropriate educational support. They need to acquaint themselves with relevant legislation and keep abreast of local and national developments in education which impact on the educational placement and provision for a child with a communication difficulty.

Useful addresses

ACE (Advisory Centre for Education)
1c Aberdeen Studios
22 Highbury Grove
London N5 2DQ
Tel: 020 7354 8318
www.ace-ed.org.uk

AFASIC (Association for all Speech
  Impaired Children)
2nd Floor
50–52 Great Sutton Street
London EC1V ODJ
Tel: 020 7490 9410
www.afasic.org.uk

ASLTIP (Association of Speech and
  Language Therapists in Independent
  Practice)
Coleheath Bottom
Speen
Princes Risborough
Buckinghamshire HP27 0SZ
Tel: 0870 241 3357
www.helpwithtalking.com

British Dyslexia Association
98 London Road
Reading RG1 5AU
Administration tel: 0118 966 2677
Helpline: 0118 966 8271
www.bda-dyslexia.org.uk

British Stammering Association
15 Old Ford Road
London E2 9PJ
Tel: 020 8983 1003
www.stammering.org

Children's Head Injury Trust
c/o Neurosurgery
The Radcliffe Infirmary
Oxford OX2 6HE
Tel: 01865 224786

Children's Legal Centre
University of Essex
Wivenhoe Park
Colchester
Essex CO4 3SG
Tel: 01206 873820 (Helpline)
www.childrenslegalcentre.com

Contact a Family
209–211 City Road
London EC1V 1JN
Tel: 020 7608 8700
Fax: 020 7608 8701
Minicom: 202 7608 8702
Helpline: 0808 808 3555
www.cofamily.org.uk

Dyspraxia Foundation, The
8 West Alley
Hitchin
Hertfordshire SG5 1EG
Tel: 01462 454 986
www.dyspraxiafoundation.org.uk

ICAN (the national charity for
  children with speech and language
  impairments)
4 Dyers Building
London EC1N 2OP
Tel: 0870 010 40 66
www.ican.org.uk

IPSEA (Independent Panel for Special
  Education Advice)
6 Carlow Mews
Woodbridge
Suffolk IP12 IEA
Advice line: 0800 0184016
Tribunal appeals only: 01394 384711
Enquiries: 01394 380518

Medico-Legal Helpline (provides information and answers questions on issues relating to special educational needs assessment and educational provision)
Tel: 0870 241 2068

National Autistic Society (NAS)
393 City Road
London EC1V 1NE
Tel: 020 7833 2299
Helpline: 0870 600 8585
www.nas.org.uk

National Childbirth Trust
Alexandra House
Oldham Terrace
Acton
London W3 6NH
Tel: 0870 444 8707
www.nct-online.org

NDCS (National Deaf Children's Society)
15 Dufferin Street
London EC1Y 8UR
Tel: 020 7460 8658
Helpline: 0808 800 8880
www.ndcs.org.uk

Network 81 (a national network of parents of children with special educational needs)
1–7 Woodfield Terrace
Stansted
Essex CM24 8AJ
Tel: 0870 770 3306
www.network81.co.uk

RNIB (Royal National Institute for the Blind)
105 Judd Street
London WC1N 9NE
Tel: 020 7388 1266

RNID (Royal National Institute for Deaf People)
19–23 Featherstone Street
London EC1Y 8SL
Tel: 0808 808 0123 (freephone)
Textphone: 0808 808 9000 (freephone)
Fax: 020 7296 8199
www.rnid.org.uk

Royal College of Speech and Language Therapists (RCSLT)
2 White Hart Yard
London SE1 1NX
Tel: 020 7378 1200
Fax: 020 7403 7254
www.rcslt.org.uk

SCOPE (for people with cerebral palsy)
6 Market Road
London N7 9PW
Helpline: 0808 800 3333
www.scope.org.uk

SENSE (The National Deafblind and Rubella Association)
11–13 Clifton Terrace
Finsbury Park
London N4 3SR
Tel: 020 7272 7774
Textphone: 020 7272 9648
Fax: 020 7272 6012
www.sense.org.uk

Glossary

Accent: a pattern of **pronunciation** that is characteristic of a particular region, or group of people

Acoustic: pertaining to sound

Active sentence: in active sentences the positions of 'agent' (i.e. the one carrying out the action) and 'patient' (i.e. the one in receipt of the action) follow the normal **word** order, for example 'the man [agent] hit the dog [patient]', with the subject of the sentence as 'agent' and the object as 'patient' (see also **Passive sentencess)**

Adjective: a **word** that is used to qualify or modify a **noun**, for example a *big* hat

Affective variables: factors relating to how a learner feels about themselves in relation to a **language** being learned, that affect the acquisition of the **language** (especially in **bilingual** acquisition)

Alliteration: occurrence of the same sound at the start of **words** in close succession, for example 'big, blue bear'

Alphabetic: referring to a system of letters

Article: in English, the **words** 'the' (definite **article**), 'a' and 'an' (indefinite **articles**)

Articulation: movement of the **articulators** to produce **speech sounds**

Articulators: general term to refer to the parts of the mouth involved in articulating **speech**: lips, tongue, roof of mouth, **soft palate**, **pharynx** and jaw

Articulatory pattern: set of instructions stored in the mind for how an individual **word** is pronounced; also referred to as a **word**'s 'motor programme'

Attachment: refers to the development of bonds between two or more people; the strength and security of an infant's early **attachments** to significant caregivers is thought to significantly influence the development of later relationships

Attention: ability to attend to a stimulus, such as spoken **language**

Auditory: to do with hearing

Auditory feedback: (i.e. of **speech**) process of hearing one's own **speech** as it is uttered; information can be used to modify **speech output** if errors are detected

Auditory processing: processing of information that is heard

Autism: neurodevelopmental condition with impaired **language**, social interaction and imagination

Autistic spectrum disorders: **autism** appears in a great range of manifestations, with levels of functioning ranging from very high to very low, thus constituting a spectrum (see also **Autism**)

Babbling: often playful sound production that precedes the development of **speech**, involving **consonants** and **vowels** in various combinations

Balanced bilinguals: **bilingual** speakers who are equally proficient in both **languages**; also termed **productive bilinguals** (see also **Passive bilinguals**)

Basic interpersonal communication skills (BICS): level of **language** and **communication** development that is usually achieved by the age of 3, that includes basic interpersonal **communication** skills with basic but appropriate **grammar** and a large **vocabulary** that is used in a largely context-dependent way

Bilingualism: referring to two **languages** (Chapter 5 contains a wider discussion of the meaning of '**bilingualism**')

Blend: (i.e. of **consonants**) sequence of two or more **consonants**, for example 'tr' of 'trip'

Blend reduction: **simplification pattern** involving reduction of **consonant blends** to just one **consonant**, for example dress → des; stamp → tam

Body language: communicative use of one's body; for example, leaning towards a speaker indicates interest in them and what they have to say

Bound morpheme: a minimal meaningful unit of **language**, serving a grammatical function, that must always be connected to another **morpheme**, for example the **plural** '-s' on 'cats'

Categorization: ability to sort objects according to their similarities and differences

Cerebellar: referring to the cerebellum, the part of the brain that plays a significant role in providing the rapid and precise **motor** control needed for **speech**; also serves a modulating function of **sensory** and **motor** impulses; has **auditory**, **tactile** and **visual** centres with many connections to other parts of the brain

Cerebral palsy: congenital disability affecting **motor** power and coordination, related to damage of the immature brain; manifestations of the disorder depend on which parts of the brain are affected; there may be associated problems in the **motor** movements of **speech**, **visual** and hearing problems, **perceptual** or **sensory** disturbances, problems with cognitive development and **epilepsy**

Child directed talk: see **Motherese**

Childhood epilepsy: epileptic seizures indicate cerebral dysfunction and usually arise from structural or physiological abnormalities in the brain; changes in behaviour, consciousness and disturbances in **motor** activity are seen; an estimated 3 to 7 per cent of children under 5 are expected to have one or more seizure, and 5 per cent of these are expected to go on to develop further **epilepsy** (cited by Lees and Urwin 1991)

Clarification request: when a listener cannot follow what the speaker is trying to say, they will sometimes make a request for clarification

Cleft palate: clefts of the lip and palate result from a failure in the fusion of these structures in utero; commonly associated with **middle ear** problems, and **speech** development is usually affected; in some children, **language** develops more slowly

Code mixing: a feature of **bilingual speech** whereby a speaker mixes elements from both **languages** within a single **utterance**

Code switching: a feature of **bilingual speech** whereby a speaker mixes elements of both **languages** across several turns in **conversation**

Cognitive academic language proficiency (CALP):   level of **language** skill involving understanding and use of higher levels of **decontextualized language** (used increasingly in the classroom as children move up the school), development of literacy skills and a developing awareness about aspects of **language** in order to derive the meaning of a **word**, sentence or **text** (see also **basic interpersonal communication skills**)

Combine words: link individual **words** together to make short phrases, for example mummy + drink → mummy drink

Communication: the transmission of a message from one person to another

Communicative functions: the uses of **communication**, for example requesting, commenting

Complex sentences: sentences that combine two or more ideas in a single **utterance** through the use of advanced grammatical structures

Comprehension strategies: see **Nonlinguistic strategies**

Conceptual categories: mental groupings of things and experiences according to the similarities and differences between them

Conjunctions: **words** that connect sentences and clauses within sentences, for example but, and, because

Consonant harmony: **simplification pattern** involving different **consonants** being pronounced as a single **consonant**, for example tiger → giger; bottle → bobble

Consonants: **speech sounds** that are made by obstructing the air flow through the **vocal tract** in some way; one way of describing **consonants** is in terms of their place of articulation, which refers to where in the **vocal tract** the constriction occurs

Constructional play: play that involves constructing something such as a tower of building bricks

Context sensitive voicing: **simplification pattern** whereby all sounds in a certain position (for example initial) of **words** are produced with activation of the **vocal folds**, producing **voice**, for example tea → dea; cup → gup

Contrastive use: (i.e. of **speech sounds**) refers to their systematic use to indicate differences in meaning; for example, the difference in meaning between 'pie' and 'buy' is signalled by contrastive use of 'p' and 'b'

Conversation: a series of communicative exchanges between two or more people

Conversational repair: recognizing occurrence of a conversational breakdown and using strategies to keep the **conversation** going

Cooing, gurgling: the stage of vocal development that starts at around 8 weeks

Coordination: joining together of two separate **utterances** using **conjunctions** such as and, because

Count nouns: **nouns** that denote an entity of which there can be one or more than one, and for which there are therefore **plural** forms, for example cup/cups, dog/dogs (see also **Mass nouns**)

Decontextualized language: language that does not rely on the immediate context for its meaning to be understood, and that communicates information that is new to the listener or reader

Delay: in development, including **speech** and **language**, results in slower development than that of peers, but that essentially follows the same pattern

Dialect: regional differences in the **grammar**, idiom and **vocabulary** of a **language**

Differentiated language systems: the separation of two **language** systems when considering linguistic processing in **bilingual** acquisition

Discourse: a stretch of spoken or written **language** extending beyond a single sentence; used here to refer to **decontextualized** spoken **language**

Disorder: of development, including **speech** and **language**; refers to an unusual pattern of development

Dominance: the **language** that a **bilingual** speaker uses with greater competence

Down's syndrome: a syndrome caused by chromosome anomaly and associated with various physical problems, developmental **delay** and variable patterns of development between individuals

Dysfluent: speech that is characterized by false starts, hesitations and repetitions, and that is distressing to the speaker or listener

Emotional abuse: 'The severe adverse effect on the behaviour and the emotional development of a child caused by persistent or severe emotional ill treatment or rejection. All abuse involves some emotional ill treatment.' (Department of Health 1999)

Emotional regulation: the ability one has to control or modulate one's level of emotional arousal

Environmental deprivation: deprivation of experiences (such as play, interaction) that would be considered normal within an individual's culture, such that a child's development is affected

Expand: to rephrase the child's **utterance**, adding more **words**

Expansion: rephrasing a child's **utterance**, adding more **words**

Expressive language: the **language** that a speaker produces, as opposed to that which they understand

Expressive vocabulary: words that a speaker uses

Feedback: information about performance that assists in modification of **output**; **feedback** about one's own **speech** assists a speaker to modify their **speech** in order to convey their message more successfully

Final consonant deletion: simplification pattern whereby the final **consonant** is omitted, for example bath → ba; cup → cu

Fluctuating hearing loss: see **Otitis media**

Form: of **language** refers to its structure, i.e. rules underlying combinations of sounds and **words**

Formulaic phrases: set phrases; children who use **formulaic phrases** may not understand or use their component **words**; use of these is usually context-bound, for example 'my turn', 'tidy-up time'

Free morpheme: **a morpheme** is a minimal meaningful unit of **language**; a free **morpheme**, for example 'cat', can stand alone

Fronting: a **simplification process** whereby sounds that are usually made in the back of the mouth (such as 'k', 'g') are produced in the front of the mouth (as 't', 'd')

Future aspect: grammatical structure/s used to express future events; for example, I'm *going to* eat this apple

Gesture: communicative movement made with the hand or other body part

Gliding: a **simplification process** whereby 'l' and 'r' are produced as 'y' and 'w' respectively

Grammar: the rules that exist in a **language** for combining **words** and parts of **words** in order to express meaning

Gurgling: see **Cooing**

Head injury: as a result of trauma either externally (penetrating head injury) or internally (closed head injury)

Hearing impairment: hearing levels that are raised relative to those of hearing people, such that acquisition of spoken **language** is affected

Hydrocephalus: a condition involving excessive accumulation of cerebrospinal fluid inside the skull due to an obstruction to normal circulation of the fluid; surgical intervention is normally indicated to create drainage so that pressure in the skull does not result in brain damage

Hypothesis testing: refers to strategies used by learners that involve testing out their understanding of (new) information, such as the meaning of a new **word**

Inflection: in English, these are the **word** endings that change the grammatical meaning of a **word**, for example **plural** '–s', **past tense** '–ed'

Initial syllable reduplication: **simplification pattern** involving duplication of first **syllable**, for example dolly → dodo

Inner ear: the innermost part of the ear that contains the organ of hearing (cochlea) and balance, and that transmits **auditory** information to the brain by way of **sensory** pathways

Input: referring to environmental stimuli, including **speech**, **language** and **communication**, that an individual receives through their senses

Intentional communication: **communication** that is goal-oriented

Interference effect: occurs when the weaker **language** spoken by a **bilingual** is affected by factors that are specific to the dominant **language**; may take place at any level, such as **pronunciation**, grammatical rules

Intonation: the rhythm and pattern of **pitch** changes across an **utterance**; in English a speaker typically uses rising **pitch** at the end of a sentence when asking a question

Jargon: name given to the later stages of **babbling**, which typically involves different sounds, which has recognizable **intonation** patterns and which might include the occasional real **word**

Joint attention: the establishment and maintenance of a shared focus of attention between two or more interaction partners

Language: the **words**, and rules for combining and using them, common to a particular group of people

Language disorder: an unusual pattern of **language** development

Larynx: see **Voice box**

Learning difficulties: cognitive impairments that affect the rate of learning and manner of learning; can affect memory, **attention**, **perception**, problem-solving and thinking in general

Linguistic: to do with **language**, or the study of **language**

Linguistic processing: the mental processes involved in receiving and formulating **language**, which are necessary to verbal comprehension and verbal expression

Listening: attending to what one hears in order to interpret its meaning

Majority language: the **language** spoken by members of the wider community, when considering **bilingualism**

Mass nouns: **nouns** that refer to a gathering or assemblage of some sort, for example milk, sky, which cannot be counted; also referred to as 'collective nouns' (see also **Count nouns**)

Mental processing: ways of attaining, retaining, considering and using knowledge in the mind

Metalinguistic awareness: ability to think about and reflect on the structure, function and nature of **language**; includes **phonological awareness**

Middle ear: the part of the ear that contains the ossicles (small bones) that mechanically transmit sound waves to the **inner ear**

Minimal brain dysfunction: see **Soft neurological signs**

Minority language: the home, or heritage, **language** spoken by members of an ethnic minority community that is different to the **language** spoken by the wider community

Monolingual: referring to one **language**; i.e. a monolingual speaker only speaks one **language**

Morpheme: see **Bound morpheme** and **Free morpheme**

Morphology: the study of the underlying rules that govern the use of **morphemes** and decomposition of **words** into component **morphemes**

Motherese: style of **speech** often used by adults to babies and young children, characterized by grammatical simplicity, exaggerated **pitch** range and concrete **vocabulary** (also referred to as 'child directed talk')

Motor: referring to movement, for example **motor** development, **motor** skills

Muscular dystrophy (Duchenne type): a degenerative neuromuscular disorder occurring in early childhood, marked by a characteristic progression of muscle weakness starting in the pelvis and trunk and later affecting the **articulators**

Narrative: **decontextualized language** that is used to tell about real or fictional events that constitute new information to the listener or reader

Negatives: grammatical structures that express forms of negation such as non-existence, disappearance, non-occurrence, cessation, rejection, denial and prohibition

Neglect: 'The persistent or severe neglect of a child (for example, by exposure to any kind of danger, including cold and starvation) which results in serious impairment of the child's health or development, including non organic failure to thrive.' (Department of Health 1999)

Neurological: to do with the normal functioning and disorders of the nervous system

Nonlinguistic: information that is relevant to **communication** that is not part of the **linguistic** signal, for example facial expression, tone of **voice**

Nonlinguistic strategies: strategies that children use to help them make sense of what is said, that do not rely on **verbal comprehension**; for example, following **nonverbal** information such as an adult's gaze or pointing finger

Nonverbal: see **Nonlinguistic**

Noun: a **word** that is used to indentify a person, place or thing

Object permanence: the understanding that children develop over the latter part of the first year that objects exist even though they may no longer be in sight

Onomatopoeic: referring to **words** that sound like the things they represent, such as 'tick-tock'

Oromotor: referring to movements of muscles within the mouth

Otitis media: inflammation of the **middle ear** due to bacterial or viral infection; associated with accumulation of fluid in the **middle ear** (normally an air-filled chamber), which impairs transmission of sound waves via the ossicles to the **inner ear**; the fluid may be reabsorbed and recur with a further infection at a later stage; this can result in fluctuating hearing loss

Output: when considering **communication**, refers to an individual's expressive **speech**, **language** and **communication**

Overextension: of **word** meaning; refers to a child's use of a **word** in a more general sense than adults' use, such as the use of 'daddy' to refer to all men

Overgeneralize: a tendency that **language** learners have to apply rules inaccurately, as in overgeneralization of the **past tense** '-ed' ending in 'wented'

Passive bilinguals: **bilingual** speakers who retain a passive understanding of one **language** but use the other **language** more actively for **communication**

Passive sentences: in **passive sentences** the positions of 'agent' (i.e. the one carrying out the action) and 'patient' (i.e. the one in receipt of the action) are reversed, resulting in sentences like, 'the dog [patient] was hit by the man [agent]' instead of 'the man [agent] hit the dog [patient]' with a subtle shift in focus to what is being talked about

Past tense: grammatical structure/s that refer to events that have taken place in the past

Perception: analysis and interpretation by the brain of **sensory** information to make sense of experiences

Perceptual processing; modification and sorting of **sensory** information by the brain, including comparing it with memories and expectations

Peripheral processing: the initial processing of **sensory** information prior to deeper processing that leads to comprehension

Pharynx: the airway in the throat that extends behind the tonsils, above the larynx and below the opening to the nose in the throat

Phonological awareness: knowledge of the sound and **syllabic** properties of words that enables children to recognize and produce **rhymes**, and to manipulate sounds in games such as 'I spy'

Phonology: the system of sounds in a **language**; how **speech sounds** are used and how **intonation** patterns of **words** and sentences are determined

Physical abuse: 'Physical injury to a child, including deliberate poisoning, where there is definite knowledge or a reasonable suspicion that the injury was inflicted or knowingly not prevented.' (Department of Health 1999)

Pitch: the sensation of sound frequency; a high-frequency **voice** produces a perception of high **pitch**

Plural: grammatical structure to indicate plurality, such as the '-s' in 'cats'

Postnatal depression: depression that occurs in a mother within a few months of giving birth

Pragmatics: the rules, or study of rules, governing the use of **language** in social contexts and in **conversation**

Preintentional communication: the stage of **communication** development prior to **intentional communication**, when children's **communication** is not yet goal-oriented

Preposition: a **word** that indicates location, for example *in* the box, *under* the table

Present tense: grammatical structure/s that refer to events taking place at the current time

Pretend play: play that involves make-believe situations, including role play

Productive bilinguals: see **Balanced bilinguals**

Pronoun: a **word** that is used instead of a **noun**, for example he, she

Pronunciation: refers to how **words** are articulated; young children have immature **pronunciation**; regional accents differ in their **pronunciation**

Proprioceptive: to do with proprioception, the receipt of information from muscles, tendons and joints, that provides information about body position and movements

Protowords: consistent and intentional use by **language** learners of idiosyncratic sound patterns, prior to the onset of recognizable **words**

Receptive language: the **language** that an individual receives, i.e. hears or sees, as opposed to that which they express

Receptive vocabulary: **words** that a speaker understands

Reduplication: **simplification pattern** involving the repetition of the first **syllable** of a **word**, such as Rowan → Roro

Referent: the 'thing' or 'quality' that a **word** or phrase refers to

Reflexive: referring to fast responses that occur as a result of internal or external stimuli

Relative clause: a type of **subordinate clause** that further specifies a thing or person (i.e. **noun**) that a speaker is talking about, for example 'The man *who is wearing a hat* is climbing the tree' is more specific than 'The man is climbing the tree'

Repair: see **Conversational repair**

Representational play: play that involves the use of real objects outside of their normal context, such as touching a brush to one's hair in play

Representational sounds: sounds that represent other sounds, for example 'moo', 'brrmm'

Respiratory system: structures involved in respiration such as the lungs, windpipe

Rhyme: occurring when two or more **words** sound the same from the last stressed **vowel** to the end, the preceding sounds being different, for example 'rabbit' and 'habit', 'bit' and 'fit'

Selectively mute: refers to individuals who do not speak in 'select' situations

Semantics: refers to the meanings of **words** and sentences

Sensori-neural hearing loss: hearing impairment from damage to the cochlea (the hearing organ in the **inner ear**), or the **sensory** pathway leading from the cochlea to the brain

Sensory impairments: problems affecting an individual's senses, most commonly referring to hearing and vision

Sequential language acquisition: pattern of **bilingual language** acquisition that involves mastering one **language** followed by learning another

Sexual abuse: 'The involvement of dependent, developmentally immature children and adolescents in sexual activities they do not truly comprehend, to which they are unable to give informed consent, or that violate the social taboos of family roles.' (Department of Health 1999)

Sign: manual gesture that has **linguistic** meaning

Sign language: a rule-governed manual **language** system that has its own **vocabulary** and **grammar**, and rules governing their use

Simplification pattern: a rule-governed process affecting **pronunciation**, whereby parts of a **word** or some sounds are omitted, or easier sounds may be used in place of more difficult ones

Simultaneous language acquisition: (**bilingualism**) pattern of **bilingual language** acquisition whereby both **languages** are acquired at the same time, i.e. from birth

Single-channelled: used to refer to the stage of **attention** development when children are only able to attend to one modality at a time, i.e. they can look at a picture but are unable to **listen** to spoken **language**

Single-word period: see **single-word stage**

Single-word stage: stage of **language** development when children use **words** one at a time, for example 'mummy'; 'drink'

Soft neurological signs: signs include attention disorders, **motor** clumsiness, **perceptual** deficits and left-right problems; there is no evidence of brain damage as such, but there is a relationship with **minimal brain dysfunction**, in that there is some problem in how the brain functions, and function can be inconsistent

Soft palate: the muscular posterior part of the roof of the mouth

Specific language impairment (SLI): a disorder involving an unusual pattern of **language** development that cannot be attributed to learning, environmental or emotional difficulties

Speech processing: all the skills included in understanding and producing **speech**

Speech sounds: sounds used in **speech**, i.e. **consonants** and **vowels**

Speech sound store: an individual's mental store of **speech sounds** that is accessed when processing **speech**

Startle response: a reflex response to sudden or loud noises manifested when the baby behaves startled (sudden movement of the eyes and body)

Stopping: a **simplification process** whereby sounds that are usually made on a continuous stream of air (such as 'f', 'v') are produced as 'stops', involving the build up and sudden release of air inside the mouth

Stress: emphasis with which a **syllable** is uttered; stressed syllables are produced with higher amounts of energy and are therefore louder, of higher **pitch** or longer duration than unstressed ones; stress is used to signal differences in meaning in English

Subordinate clause: a part of a sentence, containing a **verb**, that cannot stand alone, for example 'I need you to *play hide and seek*'

Subtractive bilingualism: loss of a **bilingual** speaker's competence in one **language** when that **language** is abruptly replaced by another

Syllable: a **word** or part of a **word** that is produced by a single effort of the **voice**; for example '*but*' has one syllable and '*button*' has two

Symbolic play: play that involves the use of objects to 'stand for' other objects, for example the use of a cardboard box as a boat

Symbolic understanding: understanding that symbols are things that 'stand for' other things; for example, both a doll and a picture of a person 'stand for' a real person

Syntax: the rules that govern the formation of sentences

Tactile: refers to the sense of touch

Telegraphic speech: name given to describe phrases consisting of two or three key **words**, such as 'mummy drink' and 'mummy drink tea'

Tense: grammatical form of a verb indicating the time of the action (see also present tense, past tense and future aspect)

Text: a stretch of written **language** extending beyond a single sentence; used here to refer to **decontextualized**, written **language**

Three-word phrases: phrases consisting of three **words**, such as 'mummy drink tea'

Three-word stage: stage of **language** development during which children combine three **words** together, for example 'mummy' + 'drink' + 'tea' → 'mummy drink tea'; can also refer to a child's level of understanding, i.e. the number of **words** they are able to follow in any **utterance**

Topic: the subject matter of **conversation**

Turn-taking: the exchange of turns between two or more people in a **conversation**

Two-word level: see **two-word stage**

Two-word phrases: phrases consisting of two **words**, such as 'mummy drink'

Two-word stage: stage of **language** development during which children combine two **words** together, for example 'mummy' + 'drink' → 'mummy drink'; can also refer to a child's level of understanding, i.e. the number of **words** they are able to follow in any **utterance**

Underextension: of **word** meaning; refers to a child's use of a **word** in a narrower fashion than an adult's, for example the use by a child of 'daddy' to refer only to her father, and nobody else's

Unitary language system: when considering **bilingual** acquisition, linguistic processing of two **languages** within the confines of a single **language** system

Utterance: the sounds and **words** that a speaker produces

Vegetative sounds: sounds made by babies in the first 8 weeks, for example sighs, grunts, squeals

Verbs: **words** that express actions, occurrences or modes of being, for example eat, remember

Verbal: referring to **words**

Verbal understanding: referring to understanding of **words**, as opposed to that of **nonlinguistic** information

Visual feedback: feedback available through what an individual sees

Vocable: see **Protowords**

Vocabulary: a speaker's mental store of **words** (see also **Receptive vocabulary** and **Expressive vocabulary**)

Vocabulary spurt: stage characterized by a rapid increase in the rate at which new **words** are learned and used

Vocabulary store: see **Vocabulary**

Vocal: refers to **voice** and using the **voice** to make sounds

Vocal development: the development of sound production by babies prior to **babbling**

Vocal folds: elastic pair of muscles situated within the **voice box** that vibrate to produce **voice** on exhaled air

Vocal play: the stage of development between 3 months and 6 months when babies produce a wide range of sounds

Vocal tract: the air passages above the larynx that act as vocal resonators, including the **pharynx**, oral cavity, nasal cavity and sinuses

Vocalization: vocal sounds

Voice: the sound produced by vocal fold vibration on exhaled air

Voice box (larynx): framework of cartilages bound together by ligaments, membrane and muscle, linking the windpipe with the **pharynx** and situated in front of the food pipe; primary function is to protect the lungs from entry by foreign particles; contains the **vocal folds**

Vowels: **speech sounds** that are made with a relatively unobstructed flow of air, and that are determined by the shape of the **vocal tract**

Weak syllable deletion: **simplification pattern** whereby the unstressed (or weaker) **syllable** is omitted, for example yoghurt → yog; biscuit → bis

'Wh'-question: question introduced by one of the question **words** 'who', 'what', 'where', 'when', 'which', 'how', 'why', which requires specific information in the response, rather than just 'yes' or 'no'; for example, 'What did you eat for breakfast?'

Word: a meaningful unit of **language** (excluding **bound morphemes**)

Word approximation: a **word** that is pronounced in a way that retains features of the adult **pronunciation**, though these may be in a different sequence, for example 'cat' → 'tak', 'at', 'ak'

Yes–No question: a question which requires 'yes' or 'no' as an answer, such as 'Did you eat breakfast?'

Bibliography

AFASIC (1993) *Alone and Anxious: Parents' experiences of the services offered to children with speech and language impairments*, London: AFASIC.

Allen, M., Kertoy, M., Sherblom, J. and Pettit, J. (1994) 'Children's narrative productions: A comparison of personal event and fictional states', *Applied Psycholinguistics*, 15: 149–176.

American Psychiatric Association (1994) *Diagnostic and Statistical Manual of Mental Disorders*, 4th edn (DSM-IV), Washington, DC: American Psychiatric Associaton.

Anderson, R. T. (1998) 'Examining language loss in bilingual children', *The Multicultural Electronic Journal of Communication Disorders (MEJCD)*, 1: 1.

Ashmead, D. H. and Lipsitt, L.P. (1977) 'Newborn heart rate responsiveness to human voices', paper presented at the Meetings of the Society for Research in Child Development, Detroit.

Baker, C. (1996) 'Perceptions of bilinguals', *European Journal of Intercultural Studies*, 7 (1): 45–50.

Bancroft, D. (1995) 'Categorization, Concepts and Reasoning', in V. Lee and P. D. Gupta (eds), *Children's Cognitive and Language Development*, Oxford: Blackwell Publishers Ltd.

Baron-Cohen, S. (1999) *Mind blindness*, Cambridge, MA: The MIT Press.

Baron-Cohen, S., Leslie, A. M. and Frith, U. (1985) 'Does the autistic child have a "theory of mind"?', *Cognition*, 21: 37–46.

Barr, R., Hopkins, B. and Green, J. (2000) *Crying as a Sign, a Symptom and a Signal*, Cambridge: Mac Keith Press.

Bates, E. (1976) *Language and Context: The Acquisition of Pragmatics*, New York: Academic Press.

Bates, E. (1979) *The Emergence of Symbols: Cognition and communication in infancy*, New York: Academic Press.

Bates, E., Camaioni, L. and Volterra, V. (1975) 'The acquisition of performatives prior to speech', *Merrill-Palmer Quarterly*, 21: 205–224.

Bates, E. and Goodman, J. (1997) 'On the inseparability of grammar and the lexicon: Evidence from acquisition, aphasia and real time processing', *Language and Cognitive Processes*, 12 (5/6): 507–584.

Bates, E., Marchman, V. A., Thal, D. and Fenson, L. (1994) 'Developmental and stylistic variation in the composition of early vocabulary', *Journal of Child Language*, 21 (1): 85–123.

Bates, E., Thal, D., Finlay, B. and Clancy, B. (in press) 'Early Language Development and its Neural Correlates', to appear in I. Rapin and S. Segalowitz (eds), *Handbook of Neuropsychology, Vol. 6, Child Neurology*, 2nd edn, Amsterdam: Elsevier.

Battle, D. (2001) *Communication Disorders in Multicultural Populations*, Burlington, MA: Butterworth-Heinemann.

Bell, J. (1998) 'How I view children's television: Fiends or friends?' *Speech and Language Therapy in Practice*, Autumn: 26.

Bench, J. (1992) *Communication Skills in Hearing-Impaired Children*, London: Whurr Publishers Ltd.

Bernstein, B. (1975) *Class, Codes and Control*, London: Routledge and Kegan Paul.

Bernstein Ratner, N. (1989) 'Atypical Language Development', in J. Berko Gleason (ed.), *The Development of Language*, 2nd edn, Columbus: Merrill.

Bialystok, E. and Herman, J. (1999) 'Does bilingualism matter for early literacy?', *Bilingualism, Language and Cognition*, 2 (1): 35–44.

Bibbings, A. (1994) 'Carers and Professionals – the Carer's Viewpoint', in A. Leathard (ed.), *Going Inter-professional – Working together for health and welfare*, London: Routledge.

Billeaud, F. (1992) *Communication Disorders of Infants and Toddlers*, Burlington, MA: Butterworth-Heinemann.

Bishop, D. (1989) 'Autism, Asperger's syndrome and semantic-pragmatic disorder: Where are the boundaries?' *British Journal of Disorders of Communication*, 24: 107–121.

Bishop, D. and Leonard, L. (eds) (2001) *Speech and Language Impairments in Children*, New York: Psychology Press.

Bloom, L. (1993) *The Transition from Infancy to Language*, Cambridge, UK: Cambridge University Press.

Bloom, L. and Lahey, M. (1978) *Language Development and Language Disorders*, New York: John Wiley and Sons, Inc.

Boehm, A. E. (1976) *Boehm Resource Guide for Basic Concept Teaching*, New York: Psychological Corporation.

Boehm, A. E. (2000) *Boehm Test of Basic Concepts*, 3rd edn (Boehm-3), New York: Psychological Corporation.

Borden, J. and Harris, S. K. (1984) *Speech Science Primer*, 2nd edn, London: Williams and Wilkins.

Bosma, J. F., Truby, H. M. and Lind, J. (1965) 'Cry Sounds of the Newborn Infant', in J. Lind (ed.), *Newborn Infant Cry*, Acta Paediatrica Scandinavica, Supplement 163, Uppsala: Almquist and Wiksells.

Brinton, B. and Fujuki, M. (1989) *Pragmatic Assessment and Intervention with Language Impaired Children*, Maryland: Aspen Publishers, Inc.

Brown, R. (1973) *A First Language – The early stages*, London: George Allen and Unwin Ltd.

Bruner, J., Jolly, A. and Sylva, K. (1985) *Play: Its role in development and evolution*, Middlesex: Penguin.

Bruner, J. (1990) *Acts of Meaning*, Cambridge, MA: Harvard University Press.

Buckley, S. (2000) *Down syndrome issues and information. Speech and language development for individuals with Down syndrome – an overview*, Southsea: Down Syndrome Educational Trust.

Butterworth, G. (1991) 'The Ontogeny and Phylogeny of Joint Visual Attention', in A. Whiten (ed.), *Natural Theories of Mind*, Oxford: Blackwell.

Butterworth, G. and Jarrett, N. (1991) 'What minds have in common is space: Spatial mechanisms serving joint visual attention in infancy', *British Journal of Developmental Psychology*, 9: 55–72.

Bzoch, M. and League, R. (1991) *Receptive-Expressive Emergent Language Scales*, 2nd edn, Austin: PRO-ED, Inc.

Cantwell, D. and Baker, L. (1987) *Developmental Speech and Language Disorders*, New York: Guilford Press.

Carlsson-Paige, N. and Levin, D. (1990) *Who's Calling the Shots: How to respond to children's fascination with war play and war toys*, Gabriola Island, British Columbia: New Society Publishers.

Carpenter, M., Nagell, K. and Tomasello, M. (1998) 'Social cognition, joint attention and communicative competence from nine to fifteen months', in *Monographs of the Society for Research in Child Development*, 4: 255.

Catts, H. and Vartiainen, T. (1993) *Sounds Abound*, Moline: Illinois: LinguiSystems, Inc.

Chace, N. (2000) *Burdened Children*, London: Sage.

Chambers, W. & R. Ltd (1998) *The Chambers Dictionary*, Edinburgh: Chambers Harrap Publishers Ltd.

Chiat, S. (1986) 'Personal Pronouns', in Fletcher, M. and Garman, M. (eds), *Language Acquisition*, 2nd edn, Newcastle upon Tyne: Cambridge University Press.

Cline, T. and Baldwin, S. (1994) *Selective Mutism in Children*, London: Whurr Publishers Ltd.

Cohen, D. (1993) *The Development of Play*, 2nd edn, London: Routledge.

Cohen, N. (2001) 'Language impairment and psychopathology in infants, children and adolescents', *Developmental Clinical Psychology and Psychiatry Paper 45*, London: Sage.

Coleby, M. (1995) 'The school-aged siblings of children with disabilities', *Developmental Medicine and Child Neurology*, 37: 415–426.

Cooke, J. and Williams, D. (1985) *Working with Children's Language*, Oxford, UK: Winslow Press Ltd.

Cooper, J., Moodley, M. and Reynell, J. (1978) *Helping Language Development*, London: Edward Arnold Limited.

Crary, M. (1993) *Developmental Motor Speech Disorders*, London: Whurr.

Crutchely, A. (1999) 'Bilingual children with SLI attending language units: Getting the bigger picture', *Child Language Teaching and Therapy*, 15 (3): 201–217.

Crystal, D. (1986) 'Prosodic Development', in M. Fletcher and M. Garman (eds), *Language Acquisition*, 2nd edn, Newcastle upon Tyne: Cambridge University Press.

Crystal, D. (1988) *Introduction to Language Pathology*, London: Whurr Publishers Ltd.

Culp, R., Watkins, R., Lawrence, H., Letts, D., Kelly, D. and Rice, M. (1991) 'Maltreated children's language and speech development: Abused, neglected, and abused and neglected', *First Language*, 11: 377–389.

Cumine, V., Leach, J. and Stevenson, G. (1998) *Asperger Syndrome: A practical guide for teachers*, London: David Fulton Publishers.

Cummins, J. (1984) *Bilingualism and Special Education: Issues in assessment and pedagogy*, San Diego: College Hill Press.

Cunningham, C. and Davis, H. (1985) *Working With Parents: Frameworks for collaboration*, Milton Keynes: Open University Press.

De Casper, A. and Fifer, W. (1980) 'Of human bonding: Newborns prefer their mothers' voices', *Science*, 208: 1174–1176.

Della-Corte, M., Benedict, H. and Klein, D. (1983) 'The Linguistic Environment', in D. Ingram (ed.), *First Language Acquisition* (1989), Cambridge, UK: Cambridge University Press.

Department of Education and Science (1988) *The Cox Report: National Curriculum Council Proposals of the Secretary of State for Education and Science and the Secretary of Wales*, London: The Stationery Office.

Department of Health (1999) *Working Together to Safeguard Children*, London: The Stationery Office.

DePompei, R. and Blosser, J. (1994) *Paediatric Traumatic Brain Injury*, San Diego, CA: Singular Publishing Group, Inc.

Dickinson, D., Wolf, M. and Stotsky, S. (1989) 'Words Move: The interwoven development of oral and written language', in J. Berko Gleason (ed.), *The Development of Language*, 2nd edn, Columbus: Merrill Publishing Company.

Dore, J. (1979) 'Conversational Acts and the Acquisition of Language', in E. Ochs and B. Schiefelin (eds), *Developmental Pragmatics*, New York: Academic Press.

Dore, J., Franklin, M. B., Miller, R. T. and Ramer, A. L. H. (1976) 'Transitional phenomena in early language acquisition', *Journal of Child Language*, 3: 343–350.

Drury, R. (2000) 'Bilingual children in the nursery: A case study of Samia at home and at school', *European Early Childhood Education Research Journal*, 8 (1): 43–59.

Duncan, D. (1989) *Working with Bilingual Language Disability*, New York: Chapman & Hall.

Dunseath, A. (1998) 'How I view children's television: Dynamic viewing', *Speech and Language Therapy in Practice*, Autumn: 27.

Edwards, J. (1979) *Language and Disadvantage*, London: Edward Arnold.

Egeland, B., Sroufe, A. and Erickson, M. (1983) 'The developmental consequence of different patterns of maltreatment', *Child Abuse and Neglect* 7: 459–469.

Emde, R. N., Gaensbauer, T. J. and Harmon, R. J. (1976) 'Emotional expression in infancy: A biobehavioural study', *Psychological Issues*, 10 (37).

Enderby, P. and Phillip, R. (1986) 'Speech and language handicap: Towards knowing the size of the problem', *British Journal of Disorders of Communication*, 21: 151–165.

Fantz, R. L. (1963) 'Pattern vision in newborn infants', *Science*, 140: 296–297.

Fawcett, A. J. and Nicholson, R. I. (1999) 'Performance of dyslexic children on cerebellar and cognitive tests', *Journal of Motor Behaviour*, 31 (1): 68–78.

Ferguson, C. (1977) 'Baby Talk as a Simplified Register', in C. Snow and C. Ferguson (eds), *Talking to Children*, Cambridge, UK: Cambridge University Press.

Ferguson, C. A. (1978) 'Learning to Pronounce: The earliest stages of phonological development in the child', in F. D. Minifie and L.L. Lloyd (eds), *Communication and Cognitive Abilities – Early behavioural assessment*, Baltimore: University Park Press.

Filipek, P. and Prizant, B. M. (1999) 'The screening and diagnosis of autistic spectrum disorders', *Journal of Autism and Developmental Disorders*, 29: 439–484.

Filipek, P. and Prizant, B. M. (2000) 'Practice parameter: Screening and diagnosis of autism', *Neurology*, 55: 468–479.

Folger, I. P. and Chapman, R. S. (1977) 'A pragmatic analysis of spontaneous imitations', *Journal of Child Language*, 5: 25–38.

Fox, L., Long, S. and Langlois, A. (1988) 'Patterns of language comprehension: Deficit in abused and neglected children', *Journal of Speech and Hearing Disorders*, 53: 239–245.

Freeark, K., Frank, S., Wagner, E., Lopez, M., Olmstead, C. and Girard, R. (1991) 'Otitis media, language development, and parental verbal stimulation', in *Journal of Paediatric Psychology*, 17 (2): 173–185.

Friedlander, B. (1970) 'Receptive language development in infancy', *Merrill Palmer Quarterly*, 16: 7–51.

Frith, U., Morton, J. and Leslie, A. M. (1991) 'The cognitive basis of a biological disorder: Autism', *Trends in Neuroscience*, 14: 433–438.

Garman, M. (1990) *Psycholinguistics*, Cambridge, UK: Cambridge University Press.

Garnica, O. (1977) 'Some Prosodic and Paralinguistic Features of Speech to Young Children', in C. S. Snow and C. A. Ferguson (eds), *Talking to Children*, Cambridge, UK: Cambridge University Press.

Garton, A. (1992) *Social Interaction and the Development of Language and Cognition*, Hove: Lawrence Erlbaum Associates.

Garvey, C. (1977) *Play*, 2nd edn, London: Fontana Press.

Genesee, F. (1993) 'Bilingual Language Development in Preschool Children', in D. Bishop and K. Mogford (eds), *Language Development in Exceptional Circumstances*, Hove: Lawrence Erlbaum Associates.

Girolametto, L., Steig Pearce, P. and Weitzman, E. (1996a) 'The effects of focused stimulation for promoting vocabulary in young children with delays: A pilot study', *Journal of Children's Communication Development*, 17 (2): 39–49.

Girolametto, L., Steig Pearce, P. and Weitzman, E. (1996b) 'Interactive focused stimulation for toddlers with expressive vocabulary delays', *Journal of Speech and Hearing Research*, 39: 1274–1283.

Gleitman, L. R., Newport, E. L. and Gleitman, H. (1984) 'The current status of the motherese hypothesis', *Journal of Child Language*, 11: 43–79.

Gloglowska, M. (2001) *Time to Talk*, London: Whurr Publishers Ltd.

Goldstein, S. and Goldstein, M. (1992) *Hyperactivity – Why won't my child pay attention? A complete guide to Attention Deficit Disorder for parents, teachers and community agencies*, New York: Wiley.

Gross, R. (1992) *Psychology: The science of mind and behaviour*, 2nd edn, London: Hodder and Stoughton.

Grunwell, P. (1987) *Clinical Phonology*, 2nd edn, London: Chapman and Hall.

Haggard, M. (1992) 'Screening children's hearing', *British Journal of Audiology*, 26: 209–215.

Hakuta, K. (1990) 'Bilingualism and bilingual education: A research perspective', *NCBE Focus: Occasional Papers in Bilingual Education*, 1. Online. Available HTTP: <http://www.ncbe.gwu.edu/ncbepubs/focus/focus1.htm>. Accessed 14 October 2001.

Hakuta, K. and D'Andrea, C. (1990) 'Some properties of bilingual maintenance and loss in Mexican background high school students', unpublished manuscript, School of Education, Stanford University.

Hall, D. (1989) 'Screening for Hearing Impairment', in D. Hall, *Health for all Children* (1996), Department of Health.

Hall, D. (1996) *Health for all Children: Report of the third joint working party on child health*, 3rd edn, Department of Health.

Halliday, M. A. K. (1994) 'The Place of Dialogue in Children's Construction of Meaning', in R. B. Ruddel, M. R. Ruddell and H. Singer (eds), *Theoretical Processes and Models of Reading*, 4th edn, Newark, NJ: International Reading Association.

Happé, F. (1994) *Autism: An introduction to psychological theory*, Hove: Psychology Press.

Harding, C. G. (1983) 'Acting with Intention: A framework for examining the development of intention', in L. Feagans, C. Garvey and R. Golinkoff (eds), *The Origins and Growth of Communication*, Norwood, NJ: Ablex.

Harris, P. (1989) *Children and Emotion*, Oxford, UK: Basil Blackwell Ltd.

Haynes, W. O. (1998) 'Single-Word Communication: A Period of Transitions', in W. O. Haynes and B. B. Shulman (eds) *Communication Development: Foundations, processes and clinical applications*, Baltimore: Williams and Wilkins.

Healy, J. (1998) 'Understanding TV's effects on the developing brain', *American Academy of Pediatrics*, May. Online. Available HTTP: <http://www.aap.org/advocacy/chm98nws.htm>. Accessed 25 July 2002.

Hetherington, E. M. and Parke, R. D. (1986) *Child Psychology: A contemporary viewpoint*, New York: McGraw-Hill Inc.

Hewlett, N. (1990) 'Processes of Development and Production', in P. Grunwell (ed.), *Developmental Speech Disorders*, London: Churchill Livingstone.

HMSO (1989) *The Children Act*, London: HMSO.

Imich, A. (1998) 'Selective mutism: The implications of current research for the practice of educational psychologists', *Educational Psychology in Practice*, 4 (1): 52–59.

Ingram, D. (1989) 'The period of simple sentences: Phonological and semantic acquisition', in *First Language Acquisition*, Cambridge, UK: Cambridge University Press.

Jaffe, J., Stern, D. and Perry, C. (1973) '"Conversational" coupling of gaze behaviour in prelinguistic human development', *Journal of Psycholinguistic Research*, 2: 321–330.

Jeffree, D. M., McConkey, R. and Hewson, S. (1985) *Let Me Play*, London: Souvenir Press (Educational and Academic) Ltd.

Johnson, C. E. (1983) 'The Development of Children's Interrogatives: From Formulas to Rules', unpublished thesis, The University of British Columbia.

Johnson, M. (2000) 'Verbal Reasoning Skills Assessment', unpublished assessment, East Kent Community NHS Trust Speech and Language Therapy Service.

Johnson, M. and Wintgens, A. (2001) *The Selective Mutism Resource Manual*, Bicester: Speechmark Publishing.

Juan-Garau, M. and Perez-Vidal, C. (2001) 'Mixing and pragmatic parental strategies in early bilingual acquisition', *Journal of Child Language*, 28: 59–86.

Kahn, A. (2000) *Craniofacial Anomalies*, San Diego, CA: Singular Publishing Group, Inc.

Kamhi, A. (1989) 'Language Disorders in Children', in M. Leahy (ed.), *Disorders of Communication: the Science of intervention*, London: Taylor and Francis.

Kingsley, E. P. (undated) 'Welcome to Holland', *Family Support Institute Newsletter*, Vancouver.

Kolb, B. and Wishaw, I. (1990) *Fundamentals of Human Neuropsychology*, 3rd edn, New York: W. H. Freeman and Company.

Krashen, S. (1981) *Second Language Acquisition and Second Language Learning*, Oxford: Pergamon.

Kugiumutzakis, G. (1993) 'Intersubjective Vocal Imitation in Early Mother–Infant Imitation', in J. Nadel and L. Camaioni (eds), *New Perspectives in Early Communicative Development*, London: Routledge.

Labov, W. (1972) *Language in the Inner City*, Pennsylvania: United Press.

Lambert, H. W. (1975) 'Culture and Language as Factors in Learning and Education', in A. Wolfgang (ed.), *Education of Immigrant Students*, Toronto: OISE Press.

Lancaster, G. and Pope, L. (1996) *Working with Children's Phonology*, Bicester: Winslow Press.

Langdon, H. W. and Cheng, L. L. (1992) *Hispanic Children and Adults with Communication Disorders: Assessment and intervention*, Maryland: Aspen Publishers, Inc.

Lansdown, R. (1980) *More than Sympathy: The everyday needs of sick and handicapped children and their families*, London: Tavistock Publications.

Law, J. and Conway, J. (1990) *Child Abuse and Neglect: The effect on communication development – a review of the literature*, London: AFASIC.

Law, J., Parkinson, A. and Tamnhe, R. (eds) (1999) *Communication Difficulties in Childhood: A practical guide*, Oxford: Radcliffe Medical Press.

Leach, P. (1997) *Your Baby and Child*, London: Penguin.

Lees, J. and Neville, B. (1993) *Children with Acquired Aphasias*, London: Whurr Publishers Ltd.

Lees, J. and Urwin, S. (1991) *Children with Language Disorders*, London: Whurr.

Lester, B. and Zachariah Boukydis, C. (1985) *Infant Crying: Theoretical and research perspectives*, New York: Plenum Publishing Corporation.

Levin, D. (1998) *Remote Control Childhood? Combating the hazards of media culture*, Washington, DC: NAEYC.

Liles, B. (1993) 'Narrative discourse in children with language disorders and children with normal language: A critical review of the literature', *Journal of Speech and Hearing Research*, 36: 868–882.

Lippi-Green, R. (1994) 'Accent, standard and language ideology, and discriminatory pretext in court', *Language in Society*, 23: 163–198.

Lock, A. (1993) 'Human Language Development and Object Manipulation: Their relation in ontogeny and its possible relevance for phylogenetic questions', in K. R. Gibson and T. Ingold (eds), *Tools, Language and Cognition in Human Evolution*, Cambridge: Cambridge University Press.

Locke, J. L. (1983) *Phonological Acquisition and Change*, New York: Academic Press.

Locke, J. L. (1993) *The Child's Path to Spoken Language*, Cambridge, MA: Harvard University Press.

Lorenz, S. (1998) *Children with Down's Syndrome: A guide for teachers and learning support assistants in mainstream primary and secondary schools*, Cambridge, UK: David Fulton Publishers.

Love, R. and Webb, W. (1992) *Neurology for the Speech-Language Pathologist*, 2nd edn, Boston: Butterworth-Heinemann.

Luria, A. R. (1961) *The Role of Speech in the Regulation of Normal and Abnormal Behaviour*, Oxford: Pergamon Press.

Maccoby, E. E. (1980) *Social Development: Psychological growth and the parent–child relationship*, New York: Harcourt Brace Jovanovich, Inc.

McDonald, L. and Pien, D. (1982) 'Maternal conversational behaviour as a function of interactional intent', *Journal of Child Language*, 9: 337–358.

Madhani, N. (1994) 'Working with Speech and Language Impaired Children from Linguistic Minority Communities', in D. Martin (ed.), *Services to Bilingual Children with Speech and Language Difficulties: Proceedings of the 25th anniversary AFASIC conference*, AFASIC, Doppler Press: Brentwood.

Malavé, L. M. (1997) 'Parent characteristics: Influence in the development of bilingualism in young children', *NYSABE Journal*, 12: 15–42.

Mandler, J., Bauer, P. and McDonagh, L. (1991) 'Separating the sheep from the goats', *Cognitive Psychology*, 23: 263–298.

Marinac, J. V. and Ozanne, A. E. (1999) 'Comprehension strategies: The bridge between literal and discourse understanding', *Child Language Teaching and Therapy*, 15 (3): 233–246.

Martin, D. (1994) 'Introduction' to services to bilingual children with speech and language difficulties: Proceedings of the 25th anniversary AFASIC conference, AFASIC, Brentwood: Doppler Press.

Mathieson, B., Skuse, D., Wolke, D. and Reilly, S. (1989) 'Oral-motor dysfunction and failure to thrive among inner city infants', *Developmental Medicine and Child Neurology*, 31: 293–302.

Meltzoff, A. N. and Moore, M. K. (1983) 'Newborn infants imitate adult facial gestures', *Child Development*, 54: 702–709.

Menn, L. (1989) 'Phonological Development: Learning Sounds and Sound Patterns', in J. Berko Gleason (ed.), *The Development of Language*, 2nd edn, Columbus: Merrill Publishing Company.

Miller, N. (1978) 'The bilingual child in the speech therapy clinic', *British Journal of Disorders of Communication*, 13 (1): 17–30.

Milloy, N. and Morgan-Barry, R. (1990) 'Developmental Neurological Disorders', in P. Grunwell (ed.), *Developmental Speech Disorders*, London: Churchill Livingstone.

Milroy, L. (2001) 'The Social Categories of Race and Class: Language ideology and sociolinguistics', in N. Coupland, S. Sarangi and C. N. Candlin (eds), *Sociolinguistics and Social Theory*, Harlow: Pearson Education Ltd.

Mogford, K. (1993) 'Language Development in Twins', in D. Bishop and K. Mogford (eds), *Language Development in Exceptional Circumstances*, Hove: Lawrence Erlbaum Associates Limited.

Mogford, K. and Bishop, D. (1993a) 'Language Development in Unexceptional Circumstances', in D. Bishop and K. Mogford (eds), *Language Development in Exceptional Circumstances*, Hove: Lawrence Erlbaum Associates Limited.

Mogford, K. and Bishop, D. (1993b) 'Five Questions about Language Acquisition Considered in the Light of Exceptional Circumstances', in D. Bishop and K. Mogford (eds), *Language Development in Exceptional Circumstances*, Hove: Lawrence Erlbaum Associates Limited.

Murdoch, B. (ed.) (1990) *Acquired Neurological Speech and Language Disorders in Childhood*, London: Taylor and Francis.

Murray, L. (1992) 'The impact of postnatal depression on infant development', *Journal of Child Psychology and Psychiatry*, 33: 543–561.

Murray, L. (2001) 'How postnatal depression can affect children and their families', Community Practitioners' and Health Visitors' Association (CPHVA) Conference Proceedings, October, 20–23.

Murray, L. and Andrews, L. (2000) *The Social Baby: Understanding babies' communication from birth*, London: CP Publishing.

Myers Pease, D., Berko Gleason, J. and Alexander Pan, B. (1989) 'Gaining Meaning: Semantic development', in J. Berko Gleason (ed.), *The Development of Language*, 2nd edn, Columbus: Merrill Publishing Company.

Newport, E. L. (1976) 'Motherese: The speech of mothers to young children', in N. Castellan, D. Pisoni and G. Potts (eds), *Cognitive Theory*, Vol 2, Hillsdale, NJ: Erlbaum.

NHS Centre for Reviews and Dissemination, University of York (1998) 'Preschool hearing, speech, language and vision screening', *Effective Health Care*, 4 (2): 1–12.

Northern, J. L. and Downs, M. P. (1991) *Hearing in Children*, 4th edn, Baltimore: Williams and Wilkins.

Olson, G. M. and Sherman, T. (1983) 'Attention, Learning and Memory in Infants', in P. H. Mussen (eds), *Handbook of Child Psychology*, 4th edn, New York: Wiley.

Pan, B. and Snow, C. E. (1999) 'The Development of Conversational and Discourse Skills', in M. Barrett (ed.), *The Development of Language*, London: UCL Press.

Paul, R. (1995) *Language Disorders from Infancy through Adolescence: Assessment and intervention*, New York: Elsevier.

Paul, R. and Miller, J. (1995) *The Clinical Assessment of Language Comprehension*, Baltimore: Brookes Publishing.

Porter, L. and McKenzie, S. (2000) *Professional Collaboration with Parents of Children with Disabilities*, London: Whurr Publishers Ltd.

Prizant, B. (2001) 'Autism spectrum disorders: The SCERTS model for enhancing communicative and socio-emotional competence – from early intervention to the early school years', seminar presented at I-CAN centre, London, June.

Prizant, B. and Wetherby, A. (1990) 'Toward an integrated view of early language and communication development and socioemotional development', *Topics in Language Disorders*, 10: 1–16.

Reddy, V. (1999) 'Prelinguistic Communication', in M. Barrett (ed.), *The Development of Language*, London: UCL Press.

Rettig, M. (1995) 'Play and cultural diversity', *The Journal of Educational Issue of Language Minority Students*, 15. Online. Available HTTP: <http://www.ncbe.gwu.edu/miscpubs/jeilms/vol15/playandc.htm>. Accessed 14 May 2000.

Reynell, J. (1980) *Language Development and Assessment*, Lancaster: MTP Press Limited.

Robinson, R. J. (1987) 'The Causes of Language Disorder: Introduction and overview', *Proceedings of the First International Symposium of Specific Speech and Language Disorders in Children, Reading*, London: AFASIC.

Roeper, T. (1982) 'Grammatical Principles of First Language Acquisition: Theory and Evidence', in E. Wanner and L. R. Gleitman (eds), *Language Acquisition: The state of the art*, Cambridge, UK: Cambridge University Press.

Rogers-Adkinson, D. and Griffith, P. (eds) *Communication Disorders and Children with Psychiatric and Behavioural Disorders*, San Diego, CA: Singular Publishing Group, Inc.

Rondal, J. A. (1993) 'Down's Syndrome', in D. Bishop and K. Mogford (eds), *Language Development in Exceptional Circumstances*, Hove: Lawrence Erlbaum Associates Limited.

Ruddy, M. and Bornstein, M. (1988) 'Cognitive correlates of infant attention and maternal stimuli over the first year of life', *Child Development*, 82: 53–183.

Sancho, J., Hughes, E., Davis, A. and Haggard, M. (1988) 'Epidemiological Basis for Screening Hearing', in B. Mc Cormick (ed.), *Paediatric Audiology 0–5 years*, London: Whurr Publishers Ltd.

Sheridan, M. D. (1997) *From Birth to Five Years: Children's Developmental Progress*, 4th edn, London: Routledge.

Shipley, K. and McAfee J. (1998) *Assessment in Speech-Language Pathology: A resource manual*, 2nd edn, London: Singular Publishing Group.

Snow, C. E. (1977) 'The development of conversations between mothers and babies', *Journal of Child Language*, 4: 1–22.

Snow, C.E. (1986) 'Conversations with Children', in P. Fletcher and M. Garman (eds), *Language Acquisition*, 2nd edn, Newcastle upon Tyne: Cambridge University Press.

Sroufe, L. A., Waters, E. and Matas, L. (1974) 'Contextual Determinants of Infant Affectional Response', in M. Lewis and L. Rosenblum (eds), *Origins of Fear*, New York: Wiley.

Stackhouse, J. and Wells, B. (1997) *Children's Speech and Literacy Difficulties*, London: Whurr Publishers Ltd.

Stark, R. E. (1986) 'Prespeech Segmental Feature Development', in P. Fletcher and M. Garman (eds), *Language Acquisition*, 2nd edn, Newcastle upon Tyne: Cambridge University Press.

Stark, R. E., Rose, S. N. and McLagen, M. (1975) 'Features of infant sounds: The first eight weeks of life', *Journal of Child Language*, 2: 205–221.

Starkweather, W. (1987) *Fluency and Stuttering*, Englewood Cliffs, NJ: Prentice Hall.

Stern, D. N., Spieker, S. and MacKain, K. (1982) 'Intonation contours as signals in maternal speech to prelinguistic infants', *Developmental Psychology*, 18: 727–735.

Stock Kranowitz, C. (1998) *The Out-of-Sync Child: Recognizing and coping with sensory integration dysfunction*, New York: Berkeley Publishing Group.

Sure Start Unit (2002) *Making a Difference for Children and Families*, London, DfES (Department for Education and Science) Publications.

Tager-Flusberg, H. (1989) 'Putting Words Together: Morphology and syntax in the preschool years', in J. Berko Gleason (ed.), *The Development of Language*, 2nd edn, Columbus: Merrill Publishing Company.

Tallal, P., Miller, S. and Fitch, R. (1993) 'Neurological basis of speech: A case for the pre-eminence of temporal processing', in *Temporal information processing in the nervous system: Special reference to dyslexia and dysphasia*, Annals of the New York Academy of Sciences, 682: 27–47.

Taylor, L. (1998) 'How I view children's television: Working with parents', *Speech and Language Therapy in Practice*, Autumn: 24–25.

Tomasello, M. and Brooks, P. J. (1999) 'Early Syntactic Development: A construction grammar approach', in M. Barrett (ed.), *The Development of Language*, London: UCL Press.

Tomasello, M. and Farrar, M. J. (1986) 'Joint attention and early language', *Child Development*, 57: 1454–1463.

Tomasello, M. and Todd, J. (1983) 'Joint attention and lexical acquisition style', *First Language*, 4: 197–212.

Tomblin, J., Morris, H. L. and Spriestersbach, D. C. (eds) (2000) *Diagnosis in Speech-Language Pathology*, 2nd edn, San Diego, CA: Singular Publishing Group, Inc.

Trachtenberg, S. W. and Batshaw, M. L. (1997) 'Caring and Coping: The family of a child with disabilities', in M. L. Batshaw (ed.), *Children with Disabilities*, 4th edn, Baltimore: Paul H. Brookes Publishing Co.

Trevarthen, C. (1977) 'Descriptive analyses of infant communicative behaviour', in H. R. Schaffer (ed.), *Studies in mother-infant interaction*, London: Academic Press.

Trevarthen, C. (1980) 'The foundations of intersubjectivity: Development of inter-personal and cooperative understanding in infants', in D. Olson (ed.), *The Social Foundations of Language and Thought: Essays in Honor of Jerome S. Bruner*, New York: Norton.

Trudgill, P. (1975) *Accent, Dialect and the School*, London: Edward Arnold.

Volterra, V. and Taeschner, T. (1978) 'The acquisition and development of language by bilingual children', *Journal of Child Language*, 5: 311–326.

Warren-Leubecker, A. and Bohannon III, J. N. (1989) 'Pragmatics: Language in social contexts', in J. Berko Gleason (ed.), *The Development of Language*, Columbus: Merrill Publishing Company.

Watson, C. (1995) 'Helping families from other cultures decide on how to talk to their child with language delays', *Wig Wag magazine*, Hanen Centre, Ontario, Winter.

Watson, C. (1998) 'Heightening the emphasis on language by blending focused stimulation with the 3A approach in the Hanen Program', *Wig Wag magazine*, Hanen Centre, Ontario, Winter.

Watson, C. and Cummins, J. (1999) 'Some things to know about children acquiring two languages', *Wig Wag magazine*, Hanen Centre, Ontario, March.

Watters, L. (1998) 'How I view children's television: Valuable videos', *Speech and Language Therapy in Practice*, Autumn: 27–28.

Weitzman, E. (1996) 'A modified Hanen program for toddlers with specific language impairment: Results of a two-year study', *Wig Wag magazine*, Hanen Centre, Ontario, Winter.

Weitzman, E. (1998) 'A summary of a fascinating book about the origins of intellectual disparity', Book review of *Meaningful Differences in the Everyday Experiences of Young*

American Children by Betty Hart and Todd Risley (1995, published by Paul Brookes), in *Wig Wag magazine*, The Hanen Centre, Ontario, Winter.

Wellman, H. M. (1993) 'Early Understanding of Mind: The normal case', in S. Baron-Cohen, H. Tager-Flusberg and D. Cohen (eds), *Understanding Other Minds: Perspectives from autism*, Oxford, UK: Oxford University Press.

Westby, C. E. (1998) 'Social-Emotional Bases of Communication Development', in W. O. Haynes and B. B. Shulman (eds), *Communication Development: Foundations, processes and clinical applications*, Baltimore: Lippincott Williams and Wilkins.

Wetherby, Al, and Prizant, B. (1989) 'The expression of communicative intent: Assessment guidelines', *Seminars on Speech and Language*, 10: 77–91.

Wetherby, Al, and Prizant, B. (1993) 'Communication in Preschool Autistic Children', in E. Shopler, M. van Bourgondien and M. Bristol (eds), *Preschool Issues in Autism*, New York: Plenum.

Wing, L. and Gould, J. (1979) 'Severe impairments of social interaction and associated abnormalities in children: Epidemiology and classification', *Journal of Autism and Childhood Schizophrenia*, 9: 11–29.

Wong Fillmore, L. (1979) 'Individual Differences in Second Language Acquisition', in C. J. Fillmore, W. S. Wang and D. K. Kempler (eds), *Individual Differences in Language Ability and Language Behaviour*, New York: Academic Press.

Index